LIVERPOOL
JOHN MOORES UNIVERSITY
AVRIL ROBARTS LRC
TITHEBARN STREET
LIVERPOOL L2 2ER
TEL. 0151 231 4022

Stress

a friend for life

Books are to be returned on or before
the last date below.

1 3 MAY 2002

D0487085

Jenni Adams

Stress
a friend for life

How to live with it,
use it and live creatively
as a result of it

Index compiled by Mary Kirkness
Illustrated by Kate Aldous

LIVERPOOL
JOHN MOORES UNIVERSITY
AVRIL ROBARTS LRC
TITHEBARN STREET
LIVERPOOL L2 2ER
TEL. 0151 231 4022

SAFFRON WALDEN
THE C.W. DANIEL COMPANY LIMITED

First published in Great Britain in 1989 by David & Charles
under the title *Relax and Unwind*
This completely revised, enlarged and edited edition published in 1998 by

The C.W. Daniel Company Limited
1 Church Path, Saffron Walden,
Essex, CB10 1JP, United Kingdom

© Jenni Adams 1998

ISBN 0 85207 318 6

The author has asserted her right under the Copyright Design and Patent Act 1988
(and under any comparable provision of any comparable law in any jurisdiction whatsoever)
to be identified as author of this work.

So far as may legally effectively be provided no liability of any kind or nature whatsoever,
whether in negligence, under statute, or otherwise, is accepted by the author or the
publishers for the accuracy or safety of any of the information or advice contained
in, or in any way relating to any part of the content, of this book.

All rights reserved. No part of this publication may be reproduced, stored in a
retrieval system, or transmitted in any form or by any means, electronic,
mechanical, photocopying, recording, or otherwise, without the prior
permission of the copyright holder.

Designed by Jane Norman.
Designed and produced in association with Book Production Consultants plc, Cambridge, England.
Typeset by Cambridge Photosetting Services, Cambridge, England.
Printed in England by Hillman Printers (Frome), Limited, England.

Contents

Acknowledgements   vi

Foreword   vii

Invitation to the Reader   ix

1   Exploring Stress   I

2   At the Heart of the Matter   17

3   Living with Stress   25

4   Creative Living   35

5   Help Yourself to Health   47

6   The Breath as a Key   57

7   Food: Nourishment or Punishment   71

8   Body Posture and Exercise   85

9   Relax and Unwind   105

Afterword   129

Appendix
     Physiology of stress   131
     Relax without tranquillisers   133
     Relax and sleep well   139
     Anxiety attack, panic and hyperventilation   140
     Basic sitting position   142
     Basic lying down position   143
     Getting up from the floor   143

Further reading and listening   145

Index   155

Acknowledgements

My love and appreciation to

My daughter Jacqui and sons Robert and David for your interest and encouragement and – for Just Being.

My dear little Mum – for, in your wisdom and fun, you taught me so much about life in living it.

Life as the process of creativity.

Thank you to

My dear friend Jo Dew for suggesting, many moons ago, that I should contact The C.W. Daniel Company with a view to publishing this book.

Kate Aldous for the charming illustrations.

Kim Faulkner for your example of how you 'sing your own song'.

Linda Cooper for advice and the table on the preparation for the reduction of tranquillisers.

Friends, teachers, students, books from past and present, for your conscious and subconscious contribution.

Foreword

Over a period of time I have been asked to provide a manual of information and techniques to support course work as well as the cassette tapes. The intention has been there for quite a while but the prompting came when I was asked to take a weekend seminar for middle management. My remit was to impart certain information, make suggestions and offer skills on stress management, general health, exercise and relaxation. An early enquiry revealed in a group of twelve people (five women and seven men) conditions of high blood pressure, overweight, stomach ulcers, chronic back pain, anxiety attack, asthma and insomnia. The conditions themselves spoke volumes and I almost felt that sharing skills and information on stress management was *adding to the stress* – as the purpose of their presence was to not only cope with existing stress but to take on more. And so, what was this all about? The stress was manifesting itself most beautifully in the physical body but the symptoms were only a smokescreen.

It became obvious to all of us at the end of the weekend that we had only just started to touch on *what really mattered*. The underlying desire was not just to show how to manage stress or raise tolerance levels, but an enquiry into ourselves on searching issues concerned with our own personal growth and development. This appeared to be moving away from the original idea of stress management and it was inevitable. I was becoming convinced of the futility of 'managing' stress without approaching the deeper issues.

When I drove home at the end of the residential weekend my head was bursting with 'Where do we go from here?' I stopped in a lay-by and started to write 'At the heart of the matter' which appears as a chapter heading in the book.

Since that time regular classes, courses, holidays and cassette tapes with the same attitude of approaching cause, core and deeper issues have both attracted and repelled people, for although it can be revealing it can also be very threatening to want to change that much.

This book is for many people. The umbrella heading of 'stress' is giving us an opportunity to meet on common ground – else could it have happened. This is for families and friends, teachers and students. It is for people who wish to find out more about their own stress in order to help themselves and others.

The following is an attempt to explore stress and why it is so much 'in the air'. There are suggestions of how to live with it, use and live creatively as a result of it, through 'minding your body' and taking very real care of yourself. There are practical suggestions on food, breathing, exercise and relaxation accompanied by well tried techniques. This is the mode of course work which also includes spontaneously 'thinking on my feet', but even then nothing is new for it is just re-discovering in different ways, at different times with different people. This is all supported by a background and reference to ancient wisdom, and closes with the afterword emphasising simplicity in our complex man-made world.

Invitation to the reader

I would like to invite you to use this book in order to define your own stress and move towards understanding its role. The aim is to allow stress to fall into its rightful place as part of life and not separate from it – part of the pattern for change and development.

The practical suggestions have all been well tried and tested personally and with many different people from all walks of life at varying ages and stages in their lives.

> *Let us be protected together and accepted together*
> *Let us not resent each other*
> *Let us be guided to each other and ourselves*
> *Let us achieve strength together and may our learning ever shine*
>   (from a Sanskrit prayer for harmony in learning)

It is said that you teach what you most need to learn. Well, I must really need to learn more about Yoga, relaxation and meditation and will do so willingly for it has helped me in my own stress and many other people with whom I have had contact. It has brought me joy and been a source of strength when the going has been tough – a blueprint and frame of reference. It never ceases to amaze me how it is always so true and so right. My love of Yoga – reading, study, research, practice, meditation, sharing and *just sitting* has brought me to this point, for which I am most grateful. My continuing quest sometimes gives me a glimpse of things as they are – not as I think, wish, want or hope but just as they are.

I shall be very pleased to hear from you – your reactions and suggestions but unfortunately cannot promise to reply. I wish you the very very best in your own personal quest.

Throughout the book please remember that you are 'on stage'. You are playing the leading role in your own play. Everyone else around you is playing a supporting role. You, in turn, are playing a supporting role to others. We are there for you – you are there for us.

> *From you I receive*
> *To you I give*
> *Together we share*
> *By this we live . . .*   (Sufi song)

1 Exploring Stress

Stress is the dynamic creative force that makes us stand, sit, run, walk, speak, laugh, cry, work, play, make love and procreate. It is the force that attracts and repels.

The work 'stress' has become fashionable and emotive. It abounds in newspapers, magazines, journals, books, training, health and educational programmes and courses, television, doctors' surgeries, business and industry. The caring professions are being swamped by the effects of it. It has become a scapegoat and umbrella heading to cover a multitude of situations – even a mark of success. It is the kind of stress that is unhealthy, unpleasant, continuous and excessive that causes distress.

The cost of stress

In society the cost of stress is often referred to in financial terms and much money is spent on stress-induced illness:

i) the cost to industry through loss of man working hours, absenteeism, diminished productivity, increased insurance and extra health charges

ii) research into the cause and effect of stress

iii) treatment and caring for people with stress-induced disease.

The cost is phenomenal at every level with physical, psychological and emotional destruction and devastation.

Stressors

Stress is a very specific state caused by external and internal stressors which evoke a response. The eminent Dr Hans Selye of Montreal studied and introduced a biological concept of stress in the 1930s. He pointed out that stress is something that cannot be avoided because it is the adaptive response of the body to any demand made of it. It is necessary to maintain life, and freedom from it occurs only after death. He suggests that it should not be avoided for it is the very spice of life.

The stress response follows a definite pattern:

i) alarm and preparation for action

ii) resistance and attempted adaptation

iii) either a) return to equilibrium or, after continuing unrelenting stress, b) exhaustion.

A physical stressor can have a specific effect, eg excessive heat burns. A psychological stressor, like isolation or overcrowding, does not necessarily have such a specific effect. However, all stressors have a non-specific effect which evokes a stress response and this depends upon the intensity of the demand and the capacity of the person to cope. The effects can be short lived or have a long-term effect even after the stressor ceases to be there.

> '*Stress is a phenomenon arising from a comparison between the demand on a person and his ability to cope*'
>
> *(Cox)*

Motivation and guide

The stress response is essential to life as a motivation and guide, but over-stimulation can become a very great health risk and much illness and disease has its roots in unrelieved stress and tension. Indeed 'rush, rush' 'pressure, pressure' 'too busy, too busy' 'deadline, deadline' can become a very fashionable way of life that can lead to a fashionable way of death, with ever increasing statistics to prove the connection.

Constructive and destructive stress

The experience of stress is as much an individual issue as your own hands and feet. There are questionnaires, indices, tables, puzzles, various 'ten point plans' for coping with, living with, fighting and befriending stress. When it comes down to it – it is your individual response which is the determining factor that can turn stress into 'distress' or 'life'.

The interpretation of a stress factor is unique to every individual. What can be constructive for one person can be destructive for another.

Constructive and creative stress is the motivating force that is required to move you from where you are to where you need to be.

Destructive stress is an accumulation of being unable to respond and adapt appropriately.

Between these two extremes there are many shades of grey on the sliding scale between movement, change and acceptance, and stagnation, rigidity, polarisation, resistance to change and lack of acceptance.

> Constructive stress is when *you* use it
> Destructive stress is when *it* uses you

The 'fight or flight' response

The body is a miracle and, when faced with danger, fear and excitement, prepares itself most brilliantly to cope.

The response to stress is a call to action 'Red Alert' and 'All systems go'.

Body and mind are prepared to cope with danger at a moment's notice. This alarm emergency action is brilliant. For example, take a hypothetical, albeit exaggerated, situation:

You are in a field enjoying a picnic and, suddenly an angry bull is running towards you. Your alarm system is alerted and you run faster and jump higher than you thought possible to get over the hedge or gate.

You collapse on the other side and attempt to recuperate. Before being able to do so fully, imagine being faced with another bull in the next field – the same alarm system is alerted and meets the demand as you run and jump and collapse on the other side into a third field when there is a further attempt to recuperate again. But there is no chance – before regaining any kind of balance another angry bull presents itself in the field, and the same alarm system is alerted and an attempt to recuperate.

However, after continuing demands are made the body eventually collapses and requires a longer recuperation period and this may have a profound and long-term effect.

The physiology of stress

The physical and mental changes produced by the activity of the nervous and endocrine gland systems are interconnected. Messages of danger, fear and excitement are received and so the story begins:

i) The muscles of the body become very tense and require more blood.

ii) The heart and lungs begin to work overtime in order to supply more blood to the muscles for action. The heart rate, breathing rate and blood pressure all soar. Hyper-ventilation, overbreathing may occur in order to supply more oxygen. The metabolic rate rises dramatically.

iii) The blood is diverted from the abdominal viscera and skin to action-stations of muscles, heart and lungs. The skin therefore begins to pale and if there are any surface wounds there is a consequent reduction in blood loss.

iv) The extra demand for blood is also met by an increase of red and white blood cells from the marrow, and the spleen releases stored blood and clotting agents. In the event of the skin being broken there is a tendency for the blood to clot more easily and therefore reduce blood loss.

v) The liver goes into action producing more glucose for fuel in the muscles.

vi) Whilst all this activity is going on the last thing that the body wants to cope with is eating and so the whole digestive system changes its nature – 'clamp down'. Internal secretions which are there to enable good digestion are immediately withdrawn as they are required elsewhere, therefore the mouth and throat dry up and the stomach and intestines too. The bladder and rectum may release any excess load.

vii) Senses are alerted in order to produce increased learning ability and perceive relevant information quickly. The hearing becomes more acute, in spite of the thumping heart; the pupils in the eyes are dilated and the eyelids open more widely in order to take in more light and see more; the sense of smell becomes more acute – hence the ability to 'smell fear'.

These are the main known reactions. More subtle ones are yet to be discovered. If you would like to know what is happening within the body in more detail, please refer to the Appendix.

Take the angry wild bull as a symbol of today's demands. For example:

- The pressure of meeting a deadline for a particular job of work
- Fierce argument over strong beliefs at work
- Unexpected redundancy
- Increased rate of inflation
- Decrease in income
- Disagreements with friends
- Running for the last train
- Getting stuck in a lift
- Illness or death in the family
- Children leaving home
- Fear of separation or divorce
- .... and so on.

No sooner does one 'angry bull' present itself than another appears, sometimes maybe two and three at a time. Although body and mind prepare themselves for action it does not always take place and frustration, anger, fear and impatience begin to accumulate, and so the inevitable build-up of stress and strain begins. The crisis system is overworked like flooding the carburettor of a car.

The automatic nervous system is unable to differentiate between various sources of arousal – being stuck in a lift or being threatened by a wild animal. Recent research into the relationship between mind and body shows that we *physically* respond in the same way whether faced with physical, psychological or emotional stress. The hypothalamus receives messages from various parts of the brain, nerve impulse and hormone secretion takes place in the same way and if *action* does not take place undischarged stress chemicals and muscle tension begin to accumulate. Under extreme, prolonged or persistent pressure the body continues to manufacture extra quantities of stress chemicals and when arousal continues the adrenal glands manufacture anti-inflammatory chemicals that simultaneously speed tissue repair but also depress the immune system. Muscle wasting and thinning of the skin may well occur. The 'fight or flight' response continues under increasing stress and pressure and if you are unable to release the accumulated energy you begin to 'stew in your own juices' and become your own worst enemy. No wonder there is an increasing interest in physical activity, health and fitness in order to burn off the accumulated excess energy.

Short-term reaction

Personal reaction to stress varies. The following is a selection of different reactions gathered from people over a period of time who have attended courses, workshops and private consultation.

Immediate physical reaction

Cold sweaty hands	butterflies in the stomach
goose pimples	yawning and eyes watering
laugh, cry, giggle	breathless
dry mouth	fidgety, restless, clumsy
diarrhoea, nausea, vomit	biting finger nails
indigestion, knot in stomach	frequent emptying of bladder
muscles tighten, tension and tremble	tachycardia (rapid heart beat)
hypertension (high blood pressure)	

Immediate psychological reaction

Freeze on the spot	take avoiding action
speechless	stare into space
mental block, miss the point	escape – get away from it all
aggressive	social clumsiness
anxious, confused, forgetful	insecure, frightened
panic	feeling helpless

Apparently positive

flash of clear thinking

brilliant artistic performance

motivation to action

best work done under stress

quick witted

able to be more positive

meet deadlines

Long-term effects

Some of these reactions are common at some time during our lives. However, an accumulation of continuing stress reaction over a period of time without regaining balance can become a way of life. A refusal to recognise or accept the messages of overloading can lead to short and long-term illness.

When a warning light shows up in the car it is necessary to attend to it rather than just disconnecting the wire so that the warning is no longer seen. Sometimes people have a blissful unawareness of the need to regain balance. At other times the awareness may well be there, but without any desire to do anything about it. There may be repeated unsuccessful attempts to do something about it – and so the long-term effect begins to accumulate. Although the original stress may *appear* to have lost its impact the reactions themselves have now become an additional source of stress.

The following is a list of effects experienced by different people over a longer period of time:

Long-term physical effects

Weak spots begin to play up i.e. old injury, arthritic joint, skin rash, eczema, asthma, chronic insomnia, constipation, diarrhoea, indigestion, headaches, chronic neck, shoulder and back pain.

Migraine

Unexpected increase or decrease in weight

Menstruation irregular or stops altogether depending upon severity of response

High blood pressure

Frequent tachycardia (rapid heart beat), breathlessness, panic attacks

Sexual difficulty, loss of libido, impotence

Sweating or crying for no apparent reason

Overeating, picking at food, loss of appetite

Dizzy spells

Unnatural fatigue leading to 'fatigue blindness'

Constantly jittery, nervy, impatient, can't sit still, talking incessantly

Long-term psychological effects

Irritability

Over-anxious and worried about the future

Over-suspicious

Depressed and feel guilty about the past

Fear of rejection and lack of confidence

Feeling of worthlessness

Can't bear to be alone

Turn in on oneself – very withdrawn

Extreme feeling of 'us' and 'them'

Difficulty in seeing another's point of view

Need to work very very slowly and can't manage too many things at once

Lose sense of reality

Inability to make decisions

Easily lose concentration

Lose sense of priority and proportion – don't know which way to turn

Lifestyle at home and/or at work

Highly competitive and over ambitious

Hard driving and hellbent on 'success'

Can't resist yet another challenge to conquer

Chronic sense of time urgency

Fitting in as many things as possible into time available

Using work as a defence against life

Hostile and ferocious towards anything or anyone that gets in the way

Hustle and bustle often counterproductive

Constantly interrupting – must have the first and last word

Feeling of fighting the world in order to survive

Familiarity with anger, fear and rage

Frightened of letting go – people, possessions and ideas

Extreme feeling of me, mine and power

Reluctance to pause and take a deep breath

Leaving no spaces in the day just to be quiet

Bored, lonely, lack of stimulation

Feeling of 'no-one to turn to'

Not enough time for other people. Not enough time for self

Too much time for other people. Too much time for self

All these and many more that you may already recognise are the 'angry bulls' of modern day society. When stress becomes a prolonged or regular feature in your life, you have very little reserve to cope. Exhaustion and breakdown can be triggered by a crisis – 'the last straw'.

Sometimes nature in her wisdom takes over to render you helpless to prevent you from killing yourself and you may be stopped quite dramatically by illness or accident. Having a heart attack or breaking a leg is definitely going to slow you down and this may be what is required for a period of re-assessment.

Ulcers, back problems and other real discomforts demand attention in your lifestyle. How else are you going to learn if you keep knocking the system – that delicate balance that is required to move through life feeling and expressing happiness with ourselves and others around us. Life is there to teach us to become aware of the fine tuning that is required.

People at risk

Any form of change is potentially stressful as change requires adaptation. Life events require time for adjustment and it is necessary to respect that as a lack of sensitivity to it can lead to a high risk toll. Big changes like separation, divorce, marriage, new job, redundancy, retire-ment, birth and death within the family, the loss of a dear one, financial crisis, traumatic physical injury and disease all require time for adjustment. Several of these changes together or within a relatively short span of time can be disastrous to wellbeing if, in the haste to get on with life as it is perceived, the need to take time to adjust, adapt and change is overlooked. Therefore everyone is at risk at some time during their lives – no one is exempt.

Your lifestyle and personality determine more clearly the risk factor, for it is *how* you adapt and change that can transform a potential hazard into an opportunity of growth and understanding of yourself and those around you.

There are plenty of questionnaires and check lists on stress and by the time you have completed most of them you are probably convinced that either you have too much or not enough stress. It is inevitable that you will sometimes experience the stress reaction, but to be in a constant state of high tension and 'red alert' is most certainly to put yourself at risk.

Balance

The human being is capable of being in states of high tension and deep relaxation and anywhere between the two. However, due to an increasing tendency to place more emphasis on the former and on speed and results it becomes very difficult and sometimes nigh on impossible to break the habit. Healthy tension is necessary to maintain life in balance.

The whole of life from microcosm to macrocosm is in a fluctuating state of change – balance between opposing forces – north and south, east and west, black and white, hot and cold, positive and negative, sun and moon, active and passive, love and fear, stress and relaxation. This is Yin and Yang at work.

Environment

The body is engaged in an incessant play to adapt to the everchanging environment in order to maintain balance. An intimate relationship exists between the physical organism and the demands placed upon it by the environment, and an increasing interest in ecology reflects that. The Chinese symbol for distress is a tree encased in lines and totally cut off from the five elements. Examine therefore not only the plant but the soil in which it lives.

External environment

The conditions that exist *outside* the body include:

temperature	air movement
chemical factors	pressure
surrounding objects	other people
oxygen/carbon	humidity
dioxide and	sound
other gases	circumstance
living creatures	area

Internal environment

The conditions that exist *inside* the body include:

temperature	body fluids pressure
water	acid/alkali balance
amounts of various substances in solution	

For continuing survival it is essential to be able to perceive change in the environment and respond appropriately. Intelligent perception is the ability to consider a situation both in the light of experience and future effect and to act accordingly. For each person there is a balance which is in a constant state of change.

We tend to be in a state of constant challenge, and a natural reaction is that of 'hurry sickness', fear, anxiety, panic, illness and premature death. It is only *part* of the conundrum to look outside ourselves for the solution. More and more pressures are being placed upon the individual to take control of our own lives. It is not the amount of stress but how you respond to it which results in where you are on the sliding scale between 'distress' and 'sheer joy in living.'

Tolerance levels

The effect of stress and the level that can be tolerated at any one time depends upon the quality of substance and the way in which you adapt at that time.

The quality of substance refers to the life force and level of balance that exists between physical, mental, emotional and spiritual states and this can be enhanced or depleted by your lifestyle.

LIVERPOOL
JOHN MOORES UNIVERSITY
AVRIL ROBARTS LRC
TEL. 0151 231 4022

The way in which you adapt relies upon your memory, perception, personality, beliefs, genetic heritage and your capacity to feel and express emotions.

There are underlying natural rhythmic cycles that cause fluctuation in tolerance levels and we are all affected by the process of birth, growth, maturity, decay and death. Premenstrual tension and the menopause, for example, can have a devastating effect. Many people are particularly prone to mood changes with the lunar cycle of new and full moon and at different seasons in the year. What can be tolerable at one time may not be so at another. Tolerance levels can fluctuate between the hour, day, week, month or year. *(See Fig 1)*

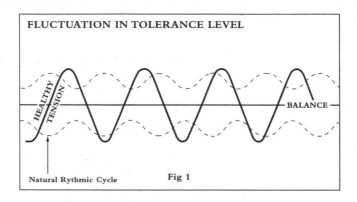

- What was not OK then may well be OK now
- What was OK then might not be OK now
- What is not OK now might be OK in the future
- What is OK now might not be OK in the future!

The quality of substance can be compared in simplistic terms with having a bank account. The current account copes with regular demands which are met with regular income to include a little in reserve for the unexpected, but this yields no interest. Fluctuating demands can be due to natural rhythmic cycles. Heavy demands and overspending lead to being overdrawn and the necessity to draw on reserves from elsewhere. It may even require a loan to continue coping with regular demands. Resources are stretched to the limit. In order to remain solvent it is necessary to re-assess the situation and regain balance of income and expenditure and reserve, and this may involve change in lifestyle. If this is not done at a time when more and more demands are being made you may find yourself no longer 'in the pink' of condition but 'in the red' – the heavy debt column of bad health. And if and when the worst comes to the worst bankruptcy may result in order to protect you and others from yourself.

Stressors test your tolerance level and ability to adapt and regain balance. *Healthy* tension is necessary to life and a continual opportunity to deal with it increases your tolerance level. *(See Fig 2)*

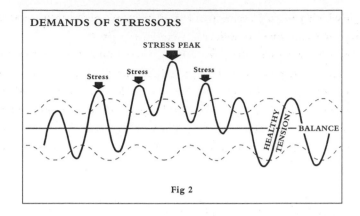

Fig 2

With more and more demands, fluctuating tolerance levels, you may find yourself juggling with life and an inability or lack of desire to bring back the balance. *(See Fig 3)* The lower

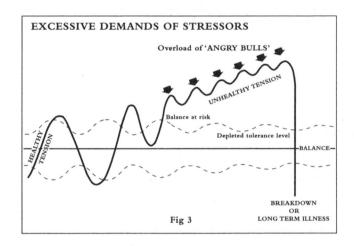

Fig 3

the tolerance level in this case the greater the experience of stress. There is an overload of 'angry bulls' and the person is at risk, maybe suffering from fatigue, fatigue blindness, frequent illness or burn-out and out-of-touch with themselves. Sleep does not seem to be enough to combat deep fatigue and your energy and life-force reserves become depleted.

Unhealthy tension ensues with such attitudes as loss of reason, inability to understand or control a situation, withdrawal, excessive time pressures and 'people poisoning'. There is a resentment from changes imposed by others, maybe even denying the problem exists. The internal milieu can no longer be maintained and breakdown is likely. Driven to the nth degree nature takes over in an attempt to bring back the balance. The person has become his or her own worst enemy.

Heart attack, angina, high blood pressure, fluid retention, reducing immunity, accident proneness, stomach ulcers, erratic breathing, aching limbs and back – and so on.

Only the individual person will know why he or she continues to test and challenge himself or herself in this way. It may or may not be obvious, and he or she may well continue to do so until it becomes a way of life, even avoiding breakdown.

Too much you burn: too little you rust

On the other hand, are you getting enough stress? With fewer external demands you need stimulus to keep the batteries ticking over, and sometimes a conscious effort to create the stimulus in order to *live* life. *(See Fig 4)*

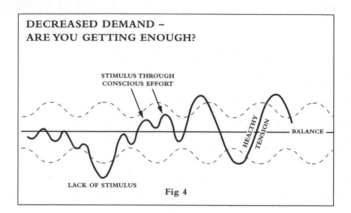

DECREASED DEMAND –
ARE YOU GETTING ENOUGH?

STIMULUS THROUGH
CONSCIOUS EFFORT

HEALTHY TENSION

BALANCE

LACK OF STIMULUS

Fig 4

With a continuing lack of stimulus, lack of interest or intentional withdrawal for whatever reason, you will experience a reduced tolerance level as well as a failure to realise your potential and use your talents as in Figure 5.

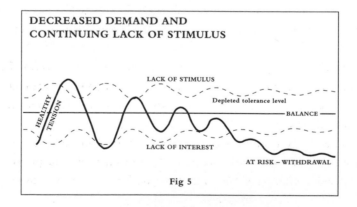

DECREASED DEMAND AND
CONTINUING LACK OF STIMULUS

LACK OF STIMULUS

Depleted tolerance level

HEALTHY TENSION

BALANCE

LACK OF INTEREST

AT RISK – WITHDRAWAL

Fig 5

Exercise

Please examine how this affects you. Prepare your own diagram like those above on a large blank sheet. Fill in the following:

i) tolerance level i.e. quality of substance and ability to adapt

ii) natural fluctuating levels

iii) label your angry bulls and stress peaks with arrows

iv) draw lines to signify your reaction and adaptation

v) are you at risk at any point?

vi) Do you recognise a need to decrease or increase stimulation and demands from stressors?

You may find that (v) and (vi) are not necessarily in accordance with each other depending upon your **awareness** of the situation and your **willingness** to act in accordance with natural laws.

vii) Do you need to reduce any of those 'angry bulls'?

viii) Can you?

ix) Do you want to?

x) Do you need more stimulation?

xi) If so, how are you going to produce it?

Doing this simple exercise at different times in the month, year and years may well highlight a variation in your need to reduce or increase stimulation.

Confronting the symptoms

Education and preventive medicine are crucial for the awareness and understanding of what stress and tension can lead to. Adopting a way of life in order to enjoy and withstand increasing pressure is a choice. If you begin to experience symptoms of stress continuously over a period of time, it is only **you** who can really do anything about it. Masking it with a smokescreen of excuses, social drugs, emotional ploys and palliative medication is just masking it.

Treating a symptom of stress is only treating the symptom and it is not dealing with the cause. Seeking out the cause can be confusing, confronting and threatening for it is sometimes far more acceptable to keep the symptom, even if this is an uncomfortable illness, than to deal with the cause.

Making an inroad towards understanding the underlying cause and source of stress is one thing – doing something about it is another. The awareness of it helps you to understand what you are really doing at the time and offers you a choice of what to do if you wish to and when.

Illness has a most useful role to play for it can be a way of coping in an attempt to maintain balance. After all, it is far more subtle to become ill to avoid a difficult situation at work or home. No reasons need be given to the boss or family – you are simply ill. Confrontation could require that you follow your feelings with action and where this is not possible the feelings remain and the body takes over for you – highly creative! It may well be that the illness at that time is the healthiest possible way of dealing with an even bigger and seemingly unsurmountable situation.

In the ancient teachings of Yoga as set out by Patanjali, man is seen as having more than one body. The five bodies are known as sheaths – **koshas** – through which consciousness functions.

Annamaya kosha is the physical body consisting of food. It covers the life force and is the poor scapegoat which manifests physical discomfort and 'dis'ease often due to an imbalance in the other sheaths.

Pranayama kosha is the etheric body or life force. It can be seen with the physical eye when a person literally *glows* with health through a beautiful experience rather than just physical health. This can also be seen by Kirlian photography. It is the level of psychosomatic patterning which affects physical change. Where the mind goes the energy goes – too little and too much.

Manamaya kosha is the lower astral sheath and seat of emotions. It is the level of perceptual awareness and both affects and is affected by behaviour and the endocrine gland system.

Vijnanamaya kosha is the higher mental sheath of philosophic ideas and intuition. Patterns are seen at this level through an overview and reviewing over a period of time. There is no remedy in Western allopathic medicine for imbalance in this sheath for it is of a spiritual nature and this is the level of 'sickness of the spirit'.

Anandamaya kosha is the bliss consciousness union with God and is unconditioned by previous experience.

Balance and nourishment are required in all these sheaths in order to experience true wellbeing. Food, sun and rest; mental, nervous and emotional food; creativity and spiritual food. The root cause of imbalance in the physical body – *annamaya kosh* – may be as a result of imbalance in one of the other sheaths and until that is attended to the physical body will continue to manifest the imbalance in one way or another.

Concentrating purely on alleviating stress and tension can lead to relief giving a false sense of security that enables you to continue to live with your illness, but still fails to deal with the root of the trouble, which may be a sickness of the spirit. Physical symptoms treated can re-appear in another way. Sickness of the spirit cannot be overcome by physical pills. Stress at work or an unhappy relationship may well be the cause of stomach ulcers but treating the ulcers does not change the situation. To remove physical stress and illness without bringing understanding and awareness to the role that it is playing is depriving ourselves of a most valuable opportunity.

> 'The cure of the part should not be attempted without treatment of the whole. No attempt should be made to cure the body without the soul. If the head and body are to be healthy you must begin by curing the mind. Let no one persuade you to cure the head until he has first given you his soul to be cured.
>
> 'For this is the great error of our day, in the treatment of the body, that physicians first separate the soul . . . from . . . the body'
>
> (Plato 427 – 347 B.C. *The Republic*)

For many centuries true healing has been practised by people guided by traditional wisdom that sees illness as an imbalance, involving the body, mind, emotions, self-image, lifestyle, relationship to the environment and spiritual beliefs.

> *'I would suggest that the whole imposing edifice of modern medicine, for all its breathtaking success, is like the celebrated Tower of Pisa, slightly off balance.'*
>
> (Prince Charles, **Speech to the British Medical Association** 1982)

2 At the Heart of the Matter

Finding the meaning in stress

Over the years, I have asked many very different people the simple question, 'Why do you want to learn to relax?' The answers have included:

'To stop worrying'
'to switch off'
'to feel calm'
'to have more self-confidence'
'because I have high blood pressure'
'because I feel tight and rigid'
'because my doctor/husband/wife said I should'
'I want to grieve and don't know how to' and so on.

In response to the question 'What do you want from life at the moment?' answers people have given include:

'time to be me'
'to cope better with people at work'
'to feel more contented within'
'people try to make you what you are not and I want to be who I am'.
'There is nothing wrong with my life – I'm physically fit, comfortably off, have a lovely wife and children and we have happy times together but there is something missing and I don't know what it is' and so on.

When clients volunteer this kind of information, we then aim to create a safe, non-threatening environment in which we can make headway through ways that seem most appropriate at the time: breathing exercises, physical movement, yoga, relaxation, meditation, prayer, visualisation, affirmation, massage, dramatherapy, reflective counselling, Bach flower remedies and reflexology.

Any one or all of these can be used in various ways. These are more than coping skills for it is more than just coping that is required. It is more to do with a recovery of meaning and purpose.

Learning and teaching

There are two ways in which we learn – either through pain or awareness. Most of us choose the former as we seem to need the experience from which to learn. Through their own awareness (maybe created through pain in the first place) parents often try to save their children from the pain of learning their own lessons. For example, just suppose there is a little girl running along a narrow high wall. Mother sees the dangers and calls out:

'Don't run along the wall dear, you might fall and hurt yourself'. The little girl continues to run along the wall and eventually falls and hurts herself badly. Where is the teacher in this case: is it the mother? the wall? the little girl herself? What *is* the lesson for the little girl. Should she stop running along walls altogether or learn how to run along the wall more skilfully without falling off?

Wherever there is pain there is an opportunity for learning. Can you equate this to the details of your own life?

When the student is ready the teacher will appear

As students of life and living, for that is what stress is about, the teacher appears in the many different guises of other people and circumstances. No one can teach you anything unless you are receptive and prepared to learn. For example, I can talk about relaxation and suggest guidelines of how to do it. You only learn when you experience and practise and then find that the learning takes place in the very doing of it – hence you have taught yourself.

Quite unexpectedly, we learn from one another. Lessons are around us all the time. The person who is happy is teaching us about being happy. The person who is ill is teaching us about being ill. The person who is in emotional pain is teaching us about being in emotional pain. The successful business person is teaching us about successful business people.

Inner reality – outer reality

Stress in our lives is nothing new, but the times in which we live are extraordinary. There is a new wave of change, a wind that is whispering across the planet, sometimes soft and gentle, often harsh and cruel. It is relentless and inevitable, presenting a challenge to the planet and everything upon it.

The age of communication in which we live brings news and information from all over the world like never before into the comfort of our homes and fireside. The space race continues; science advances like never before; big powers confront each other to threaten the whole world; financial and economic structures go haywire, fast moving and changing fashions of consumer society gobble up energy; the family unit is changing its nature, for separation and divorce are no longer unusual; more and more people are living alone; unemployment, automation, redundancy, early retirement, competition to live, let alone secure a job. Disease is on the increase – cancer, AIDS, 'new' viruses, coronary heart disease and so on. We are forced to notice the stresses all over the world and cannot pretend they do not exist. It is as though we are walking a tightrope in order to live from day to day.

Living in an age of high exchange we have to learn to change and adapt at speed in order to survive and survive well.

Old values are becoming obsolete. Big industry begins to rock and is forced to look to the wellbeing of the individual and the move is towards **people** as the bottom line as well as **profit**.

In dealing with our own individual situation it is as well to keep it in the context of the whole in order to bring about some semblance of continuity and sanity in what can appear to be a very fragmented, insane and insecure world. The unrest that abounds in the world manifests at our own individual level. We can no longer separate ourselves from it. We are forced to look to ourselves through the mounting stress experienced at an individual level. The essence of nature is to harmonise any imbalance. As human beings out of touch with nature we have become stuck in our ways of thinking and living and have forgotten to listen for the soft whisper of change. Change we must in order to survive and survive well.

There is a gradual disappearance of many animal species due to civilisation. The planet is being desecrated from the rain forests to the North Sea.

This planet is our home. How can we possibly think that we are separate?

We seem to have become so obsessed by existing and succeeding that we have forgotten how to *live* and *be*. There is a tremendous sense of loss, no matter how much material gain. The natural reaction of complementary medicine, health fitness, leisure industry, personal growth, meditation, creative therapies and finding out about ourselves is an attempt to find out who we really are, what we are about and why we are here.

As human beings we are only a part of our environment. When the environment or anything else in it changes it is necessary for us to change in order to maintain balance. This also demands that we attend to the environment in order to survive. Stress presents itself in the quickening heartbeat and in many uncomfortable physical ways, traumatic relationships, and so on. As we are forced to deal with our own stress we also attempt to keep abreast of the times that are propelling us forward at tremendous speed. This is not only the stress of the natural cycle of birth, maturity, decay, death and rebirth. The polarities that are manifesting are those of increased violence and a deep seeking for peace with both forces at work not only internationally but nationally and locally in our own towns, villages and homes. There are the polarities of an increase in the 'new' epidemic diseases and the swing towards health and wellbeing. The stress that we experience now is the quickening that is of one energy and one source but manifests either positively or negatively, in love or fear, peace or violence. It is the powerful negative experience that propels us forward to the positive. For example, as a result of life-threatening disease or nervous breakdown people are often exposed to the most wonderful therapies which shine a new light on life. The apparently negative experience has become the catalyst for change. Many people who have experienced these very threatening situations have often been heard to say that it was the best thing that ever happened to them for it awakened that which lay sleeping – a different reality.

Crisis and opportunity

With the wave of disaster and destruction there is new hope. In the crisis there is the opportunity – the transformative quality available to us if we choose to take it. The time in which we live is also wonderful, exciting and challenging. The disasters are opportunities to really transform ourselves, our environment and our world. But we must first start with ourselves.

Through communication, pop music and concerts, communities, craft workshops, small business, business focusing on the wellbeing of the individual, Greenpeace, Friends of the Earth, One World, Wild Life, Amnesty International and many other groups and organisations, more and more people are turning to find a more acceptable way of life. Many ancient teachings have a new relevance.

> *'Wherever there is a withering of the law and an*
> *uprising of lawlessness on all sides,* then
> *I manifest Myself.*
> *For the salvation of the righteous and the destruction*
> *of such as do evil, for the firm establishing of the*
> *Law, I come to birth age after age.'*
>
> *(Bhagavad-gita)*
>
> *'And don't be troubled when you hear the*
> *noise of battles close by and news of battles far away.*
> *Such things must happen, but they do not mean that the end*
> *has come. Countries will fight each other; kingdoms*
> *will attack one another. There will be earthquakes everywhere,*
> *and there will be famines. These things are like the*
> *first pains of childbirth.'*
>
> *(The Gospel according to Mark 13. 7–8)*

Success and failure

There is pressure in our society to be healthy, good looking, successful, have material wealth, a happy marriage and children who have the same attributes – and all seen to be coping with life. Society tends to see people who succeed and fail – good and bad. The very word 'success' stimulates its supposed opposite of 'failure' and even before we start school there is a reward attached to success. For the person hellbent on success, the phrase 'I'll do it if it kills me' could well be true. Alternatively, the risk of not succeeding can be so great that the easy option is to fail. 'A symptom of the moral flabbiness born of the exclusive worship of the bitch goddess SUCCESS' wrote William James. So we need to remember that it's OK to make mistakes and daring to fail can, in fact, lead to success.

Coping and not coping

Society also expects that we cope in meeting demands made upon us. When we do not meet these demands it may well be seen that we are not coping. Everyone is coping, it is just that people cope in different ways.

Illness is one way of coping – it is a statement made by the psyche on a subtle level that all is not well and there is an attempt to re-establish a harmony of the whole. Becoming ill is not an isolated incident. In our naivety we continue to 'treat' the physical body without concern for its root cause.

Sometimes it is far too difficult to consciously change or do what is expected of us, whether by others or ourselves. Becoming ill is an alternative route. The message is subtle and usually met with the 'rewards' of comfort, caring and love. This can allow the person to take time out, recoup, change route or contact the source of the imbalance. Distress, tension, anxiety, illness can become a way of life for some people for it is their way of coping with life with all its tragedy, turmoil, beauty and wonder.

> *'Heal, if you can, with respect, but do not tamper wastefully with disease within a person's destiny. The ostensible result of such cures will be living corpses, individuals who no longer have access to spiritual power because they have bought off a serious disease with their souls.'*
>
> (Richard Grossinger *Planet Medicine*)

Just listen to how a woman in her mid-fifties with a progressive disease described the pain in her lumbar spine: 'I just ache all the time. It hurts so much – if only it would stop for a moment. And when I wake up in the morning it is still there.' I asked her to look closely and deeply at what had been in her life for so long to manifest in the body in that way. What has she been lumbered with? What has been aching inside for so long that she has been unable to express, accept or do anything about?

In searching, she found a realisation and recognition that the pain of other levels was literally 'sitting' in her body. She is well aware of the fact that, at the moment, it is more appropriate and acceptable to have the illness than to communicate with the people and situation concerned. The source of the discomfort has been identified through the trauma of illness and is beginning to bring a different reality and understanding to life about choice on a subtle level. The diagnosis of the disease, although a shock, was still easier to bear than working with the cause.

Being well and healthy does not only mean absence of disease – it also includes taking responsibility for any illness we decide to have.

Know stress – know life

Stress creates the potential for change. With a low stress factor life is dull, stagnant, lacks vitality and driving force. Stress needs to be known for it is the motivating force that creates more life.

Maybe Goldilocks had it right when she established what was *just right* for her – *not* the hard chair, *not* the soft chair but the chair that was *just right*. Stress gives us the opportunity to know about ourselves and life – to find out how much life we can stand, to test our fears and self-imposed boundaries and limitations, to guide us to our own levels and realise our value and talents. Stress is the best possible teacher.

Change

Change is the very essence of life. A snake sloughs off its old skin, the unborn baby emerges from the mother's womb, the baby chick cracks open its own shell – none are without effort and struggle which essential to change, to grow, to shift from one way of living to another.

Anxiety does not mean that there is something wrong with you, but that there is something in your life that has to be dealt with *by you*. It may mean making changes within yourself and your environment, relationships, where you live, work, the job that you do and so on. These may have been with you for a long time, things about which you may never have been particularly happy or that have become intolerable over a period of time even though they had appeared to be right at one time. Covering the situation up with another problem is not really dealing with the basic dissatisfaction.

Problems

To have problems is a true sign of being alive – the bigger the problem the more life there is to live. A problem is a set of circumstances that threatens your wellbeing. These circumstances include yourself, other people and things. Solving your problems is sometimes possible and sometimes not. Changing yourself is *your* choice. Changing other people and things is not so easy. The problem you consider to be external is not necessarily so. It could be that *you* are the problem and *you* are its solution. Define the problem first rather than fighting the symptoms. There are various alternatives you could discover:

i) blame others, create an illusion and make yourself feel better

ii) wear a 'horse-hair' shirt, become a martyr and enjoy the added attention from friends and family 'Oh you poor thing isn't it awful'

iii) adopt the 'why me' attitude

iv) spread unhappiness through the family with blame and self pity

v) make your doctor's life a nightmare

vi) keep 'shopping around' for the best advice, enjoying the agony without real intention of doing anything about it.

Does happiness really lie in getting what we want? Is it really freedom from pain and suffering? We go to the limit to dodge pain but it is the only instrument sharp enough to prune away the excess dross that leads us to our finer qualities.

Crisis, exhaustion, illness and breakdown can be cathartic. However, you can still choose to repeat the pattern if you wish if you have not got what you really need out of the process. The doctor prescribes the medicine but nature does the healing, and the essential ingredient is the belief and desire of the patient to improve. The ancient *Upanishads* refer to this attitude – 'When the mind rests steady and pure then whatsoever you desire those desires are fulfilled'. It is the steadiness and purity of the mind however that are the first requirements.

Stress plays a most important role. If it is masked by treating the symptoms and/or taking tranquillisers, it may well repeat itself in the same or different form. The disappearance of physical symptoms may be just that. Real health is the discovery of an enhanced reality and new consciousness that comes from within and not from an external source.

Ingredients for positive change

   i) understand the *cause* of stress rather than treat the symptom

  ii) face the *truth* and accept your own situation

 iii) have an *awareness* of the possibility of *change* or *acceptance*

 iv) have a *desire* to change or accept

  v) *act* upon that desire.

The chapters that follow offer skills and ways of living with, using and enjoying stress in order to improve the quality of your life.

Accept, adjust and achieve

There are certain situations which cannot possibly be changed. Here you have a choice – either accept or not accept. The act of simple (but not always easy) acceptance changes your attitude from fighting against the situation to allowing it with grace. Accept, adjust your attitude and behaviour to that acceptance and then start to achieve some peace of mind. If your situation is intolerable can you do something about it? Can it be changed? If so, start to do so even in the smallest way.

If your problem cannot be changed can *you* change towards it? Can you change your attitude to it? Can you accept it? Be still with it for a while, be gentle with yourself and think about accepting it. You may begin to feel a little lighter as the burden appears to lift even though it is still there. Can you adjust to that acceptance? In accepting, take your time, allow yourself to adjust slowly and easily. This is no easy task and yet once you have truly accepted you will find that the adjustment automatically slips into place with a new way of life dawning. There will be times of reminding yourself of your acceptance and adjustment. Changing your lifestyle means changing old habits too. Old habits often re-present themselves for that is their nature. You are then being given an opportunity to notice them and re-affirm your acceptance and adjustment.

Live one day at a time – in this place, at this time and with these people here and now. Plan for tomorrow but live until bedtime.

Pastor Friedrich Christoph wrote about sweet surrender, the source of tranquillity and peace of mind:

> *'God grant me the*
> *Serenity to accept the things I cannot change;*
> *Courage to change the things I can; and*
> *Wisdom to know the difference.'*

3 Living with Stress

Cope and survive

It is necessary to cope in order to survive. *How* you cope determines whether you just manage to survive and withstand pressures or live life and use the pressures as motivation and guide to make positive choices. 'Coping with', 'suffering from' and 'being under' stress have negative connotations. Stress is life! 'Alive with' and 'experiencing' put you firmly in a positive position for change, *using* the stress in your life. Let us all do what we can to remove the management of stress *out of the doctors' surgeries* and *into life*. In the 4th Century BC, Plato was already advising:

> *'And it's disgraceful too to need a doctor not only for injury or regular disease, but because by leading the kind of idle life we have described we have filled our bodies with gases and fluids, like a stagnant pool and driven the medical profession to invent names for our diseases, like flatulence and catarrh. Don't you agree?'*
>
> ('Physical Education' in *The Republic*)

The Nobel prize for Physiology and Medicine 1987 was awarded to Dr Susuma Tonegawa who found that the body began to produce billions of cells in response to possible attacks even before germs, viruses and spores were involved. It is not by chance that there is great interest in the immune system and a continuing increase in the attainment of good physical health for it is the innate wisdom and psychic side of the body's immune defence system that leads us to this to prepare us for the increasing demands. This fashionable craze for health and stress-proofing manifests at all levels to suit all pockets, and we are all offered a wonderful opportunity to get into shape physically and mentally.

Stimulation and de-stimulation

Rapid change creates high stimulation and in order to reduce human damage it is necessary to de-stimulate and attend to your environment by 'fine-tuning' it. Some of the ways in which this can be done are by giving your attention to life-changes and stability, monitoring information, structure, freedom, decisional stress and your spatial requirements.

Life-changes and stability

Change is the nature of life and in itself can be part of the environment. Dr Thomas Holmes and Richard Rahe of the University of Washington School of Medicine have researched this fact and produced a 'Life-Change Units Scale' that measures the amount of change that an individual has experienced in a span of time. Different kinds of life-changes carry different impact. For example, the death of a spouse, divorce, getting married and moving house can hardly be compared and yet all demand many changes of varying degree. The more fundamental the change, whether imposed or through choice, the higher demand there is on your capacity for change. Our rapidly evolving society, therefore, with all the changes that are demanded, has a correspondingly high risk factor on the individual.

Life-changes are happening all the time. Some appear to be good and others not good but they all require adaptation. Marriage, separation, divorce, children leaving home, illness, accident, new car, holidays, promotion, redundancy, retirement, moving house, changing jobs, unemployment, menopause, birth, growth, maturity, decay and death – all require considerable adaptation. Sometimes several of these happen together and your tolerance level will be truly tested. When you are at a low ebb, your weak spots start to play up. You 'catch' the cold or virus that is going around as a result of your immune defence system's inadequacy to cope with the flood of demands of change that come from testing the nervous and endocrine systems.

Overstimulation and facing rapid change can lead to confusion, extreme irritability, tension, anxiety, fatigue, distortion of reality, disorientation and emotional withdrawal. We can, to an extent, make a life-change forecast and prepare to adapt or limit those changes before we are overcome by them. This is not suppressing change but becoming more aware of it and anticipating it – short, medium and long-range forecasting. A life-change forecast can help to guide you away from overloading.

Take as an example a young man of twenty who is moving away from home for the first time into his own flat. He is starting a new job and is also taking driving lessons. He could anticipate having to adapt in the following way:

- moving away from the familiar and protected environment where he has been looked after since he was born – leaving his parents, brothers and sisters

- doing his own shopping, washing, cleaning, cooking and clearing up. A change in financial arrangements to support himself totally, together with the extra pressure of his own home maintenance

- new routines of the job, new travelling arrangements to and from work and home

- learning the new skill of driving and expecting to take a test.

These may all appear to be good and exciting – but they all require adaptation. It can be a great help to make sure there is stability in other areas of life, such as:

- stable relationship with steady girlfriend

- familiarity of same peer group

- regular meetings during the week at fixed times with friends, family and/or sports fixtures

- getting up at the same time every morning to go jogging, swimming or a regular time of exercise and meditation

- wearing familiar 'old favourite' clothes and even using the same cup and plate every morning.

Take another example, a woman of fifty, happily married whose husband is a business executive aged fifty nine. Between them they have a son of twenty who is just about to leave home to go away to work and another son of eighteen who is preparing to go to university. Her widowed mother can no longer look after herself in her own home. Her husband's parents have just moved to a 'home of their dreams' by the sea over three hundred miles further away. They have a married daughter who is just about to have her first baby and wishes to continue working.

This woman can expect:

- changes within herself – menopausal and hormonal affecting her physical wellbeing and emotional stability
- her husband's retirement may mean more time together with him and adjustment at home
- the excitement of her first grandchild could also mean babysitting and caring for the baby when her daughter is ready to return to work
- to let go of her two sons as they leave home; and also to deal with their return with friends and loads of washing and being fed for spasmodic periods
- caring for her mother and the decision whether to welcome her into the family home which may involve 'budging up', building an extension, moving home, changing relationships within the home, or else exploring the idea of finding somewhere where her mother can be cared for by other people and all that that entails
- to be making long journeys to visit in-laws and to have them to stay for longer periods than before.

This is **not** the time to have a long vacation, take up a new interest or recarpet the house! Keeping a regular interest and enjoying quiet times together with her husband could be a very stabilising influence.

There are certain changes that cannot be anticipated like sudden illness, accident, death of a near one and unexpected redundancy etc.

However, with a number of big changes as *known* quantities there needs to be a safety margin within the tolerance level when you spread yourself very thinly. The 'straw that breaks the camel's back' need only be something quite minor to shift the balance from *just coping* to exhaustion or breakdown.

Familiar ritual also plays a vital role in ensuring our stability:

- fixed *festivals* and national holidays
- end of the *tax year* in April
- the same dinner at *celebration times* such as turkey at Christmas
- the same place for a *holiday*

- the opening celebration of particular *sports seasons*
- having a regular dinner *get-together* with friends or family
- taking the dog for a *walk* at the same time
- having a *cup of tea* at the same time
- regular time for *prayer*, *meditation* or *study* during the week
- daily and weekly *personal discipline*.

Take a look around you and you will see people who are always changing – houses, jobs, partners, exciting holidays and so on. If they are thriving, take a closer look to see what the stabilising influence is.

You might like to anticipate your own life-changes and involve the following:

- change in structure of your *relationship* to your parents, children, partner, friends and changes for them which affect you
- your *physical wellbeing*
- *occupation* – study, self-employment, promotion, part-time, transfer, redundancy, retirement
- *home* – move, change of use, extension
- financial *income* and expenditure
- *way of life* – social structure, leisure, travel, car, holiday.

To make your own Life-Change Forecast list the anticipated changes which affect you directly and indirectly in the following timespan:

a) *short range* – one month to one year

b) *medium range* – one year to five years

c) *long range* – five to ten years.

Use that information to gauge:

a) *how much stability* you need to create in your life

b) *what kind of stability* you require

c) *set about creating it now*.

Monitoring information

The five senses of smell, taste, touch, hearing and sight are the ways that you take in information. You can choose to smell a flower, taste an apple, stroke the dog, listen to a concert or look at a good book and so on. However, you do not necessarily choose to smell the diesel and oil fumes, taste additives, be jostled around in the underground, hear grim news, loud traffic and violence on the television.

You can make a conscious effort to reduce information overload:

- reduce trivia by writing down things you really wish to remember
- regulate the *amount* and *content* of television, radio and music and monitor the volume
- regulate your exposure to artificial, flashing, flickering and coloured lights
- make sure you have time alone to be with yourself. This means being disciplined and truthful to yourself and other people. It may mean literally shutting your front door and taking the telephone off the hook.

There is a great deal that cannot be avoided but there are ways that you can make adjustments. Conscious awareness of subliminal intrusive stressors may be all that is necessary to do something about them.

Structure, freedom and decisional stress

Decisions are being made all day by everyone but when there is an overload of information and decision making there is a tendency to postpone, to 'pass the buck' or to freeze up altogether. Subconscious effort to let other people make decisions for us happens: 'You decide for me' in response to 'What shall we have for dinner?' 'Where shall we go on holiday?' 'What shall we do tomorrow?' 'What would you like for Christmas?' and so on. Even an invitation to learn a new skill or game is just too much, and as we jokingly opt out we can be displaying an underlying need to cut off.

Structure and form are necessary in order to maximise our creative potential. Too much structure and planning limits the ability to adapt appropriately and you can become rigid, have fixed ideas, become bored, boring, fearful of change and in a rut. With too little structure and planning you can use up valuable energy in simply getting through the day. 'There is no more miserable person', wrote William James 'than one for whom the lighting of every cigar, the drinking of every cup, the beginning of every bit of work are subjects of deliberation.'

i) Create a structure for yourself that copes with the daily trivia effectively so that there are fewer minor decisions to make, about routine times, places, clothes and food. *Limit* your time each day to *specific* hours for telephone messages in and out, letter writing, shopping, planning, meetings, lunch and so on.

ii) If you have too much structure in your life, introduce learning a new skill involving decisions.

iii) Delegate where appropriate and allow others to make decisions; don't be afraid to share the routine in order to share the freedom.

iv) Let go some responsibility if you want more time to maximise your freedom, creativity and potential.

Spatial requirements

The proximity of other people is a study in itself known as proxemics, based on man's spatial requirements of territory and zone. Different situations demand an appropriate and safe distance. Meeting a long lost friend, walking with a neighbour, meeting people for the first time at a party, attending an interview for a job, and giving a talk – all have their comfortable and threatening areas. Intrusion and pollution from other people invading your safe space is known as 'people poisoning'. Animal instinct comes to the fore in the protection of that space in order to maintain a sense of self.

i) Imagine an air bubble around you as a protection of yourself.

ii) Treat it with respect as it is also a form of protection.

iii) Be very aware of its presence with regard to the proximity of other people and things – who it is, what it is, when it is, where it is, how it is and why it is and make conscious decisions based on your feeling of self preservation.

iv) Have respect for other people's air bubbles too.

Time management

There is plenty of time for everything that *needs* to be done. What matters is how you use the time. It is not necessarily a case of finding more time but choosing to use it in a different way. Time management is more to do with managing yourself in any given period of time. 'If you want something done ask a busy person' refers to the person who meets deadlines and always arrives on time.

'Where does time fly?' we say as we struggle against it, changing night into day with working hours cutting across natural rhythms. We wonder why we feel so pressurised and stressed by time and then race to have 'time off' in order to fill that time too. But the seasons cannot be hurried and so it is no wonder that we feel the need to remind ourselves of the universal pulse with our innate need to resort to Mother Nature's rhythm. John Masefield in his poem *Sea Fever* refers to this basic drive:

'I must go down to the seas again for the call of the running tide
Is a wild call and a clear call that may not be denied.'

As well as resorting to the natural rhythm for refreshment we could do well to recognise it and live by it more. Accept that *you too* have your mood swings of highs and lows, that you ebb and flow, that there are fallow periods, resting times, waiting times, times of transition and frustration, of action and retreat.

However, if you have the notion that today is a day of rest for you, it may not fit very well into your busy man-made week of office, shop, meetings, train and meal times. We can become 'out-of-step' with ourselves when we forget and work against natural rhythm. Sometimes we follow our natural cycles, it feels as though we are working against ourselves, and our thinking process can think it knows best. In fact we are short-changing ourselves when we overlook the universal rhythm that abounds both around and within us. There is the time and space of the ages and planets. The rhythm of the sun and moon affects all things and day follows night as night follows day relentlessly. The four seasons come and go and so too the monthly cycle, nine month gestation period of the foetus in the womb, heart beating, breathing in, breathing out and the clock ticks by the second, minute, hours, days, weeks, months and years. The internal clock in the pineal gland of the swallow sends it flying over vast continents. Many a seed is planted with the new moon to catch the impulse of the lunar cycle. To start a project with a new moon and aim to complete with a full moon catches that same impulse.

> 'To every thing there is a season, and a time to every purpose under the heaven;
> A time to be born, and a time to die; a time to plant, and a time to pluck up that which is planted;'
>
> (Ecclesiastes III v 1–2)

How can we think we are separate from the universal pulse when we are part of it? And yet civilisation teaches us that we can manage, save, take, lose, fight, and race against time, which is referred to as an enemy, from our own making. Surely what we are doing is becoming our own enemies.

Just as there are four seasons, there are four parts to the breath – flowing in, holding in, flowing out and holding out. Energy follows the same pattern. There is a natural time to draw in, be still, refresh, build up reserves and prepare for action; a natural time to let go and be in full-swing and busy; and a natural time to wait, before drawing in again. At the beginning and end of each stage there is a period of transition and change. There are two stages in particular that can lead to confusion. At the end of the period of stillness, just before action, you may feel full of anticipation, excited, nervous and hesitant. It is as though you are 'ready for the off' but don't necessarily know where to go and what to do. You could know precisely what you are going to do but have difficulty in being still and feel very impatient. Similarly at the end of the period of waiting and lying fallow there is a feeling of frustration, impatience and real resistance to waiting – wanting to get going again. These are stages to be recognised and used.

Waiting, in particular, can be most valuable in order to let patterns evolve in their own time. 'Just wait' has a profound wisdom. A time of waiting and stillness is natural before action in order for that action to be most fruitful. So instead of becoming anxious, accept it as a time to build up. The transition stage of birth is a time of great frustration and the mother often thrashes around impatiently and angrily before the final stage when all her energy is required to help her baby arrive into the world. Similarly there can be a stage of frustration, annoyance and impatience just before a new phase of your life, a celebration, special occasion or venture. This stage of holding back and building-up is required in order to release your full power.

Using your unique cycles

Each part of the twenty-four hour cycle has its own nature. For example, very late at night through to the early part of the morning are the hours of high creativity – the time that the musician, poet and writer burn the midnight oil. It is also known as the hour of the wolf – a time of reaching the depths of despair. The same creative force is flowing and is determined by the individual reflection.

If you have a natural tendency to being an 'early worm' or 'night owl' and are full of energy at a particular time of day or night — then *use* it. Similarly if you find that you lack energy at a particular time, use that too and rest. Trying to work against that natural energy pattern, or allowing yourself to be swept along by someone else's, can be not only very tiring but waste a very valuable resource — that of your own prime time.

Accept and befriend your own pace and rhythm. Get in step with yourself and in your own stride. You can be of great value to yourself and others in this way.

> *'If a man does not keep pace with his companions, perhaps it is because he hears a different drummer. Let him step to the music he hears, however measured or far away.'*
>
> (Thoreau)

Ninety minutes

Within the cycle of breathing there is a tendency for one nostril to have dominance over the other for a period of approximately ninety minutes followed by dominance of the other. This proven fact highlights the balancing act that exists within the autonomic nervous system — that of the *activity* of the sympathetic nervous system and the *passivity* of the parasympathetic nervous system — natural times to be active and passive.

The span of one and a half hours plays an interesting role within the twenty four hours. The ideal time for a meeting, a lesson and any activity is one and a half hours. Beyond that, unless there is a shift of attitude, energy wanes. You may be familiar with listening to a lecture which lasts for two hours or more and have the experience of losing concentration and 'opting out'. Use this fact to manage your day, changing the nature of what you are doing approximately every one and a half hours and you will find great benefit in the satisfaction of getting things done.

Time sharing

Ancient Greek wisdom suggests that the twenty-four hour day can be used to greatest advantage if it is divided equally between work, rest and recreation. There are one hundred and sixty-eight hours in every week which, if divided equally into three, gives fifty-six hours each for work, rest and recreation.

Here is a workshop where the input is from you. Its usefulness is up to you, how you use it and what you find out about yourself for you.

i) Write out three headings — Work, Rest (including sleep), Recreation.

ii) Write out underneath each heading a list of the things that are included in your typical week. You may find that it is your attitude that determines which heading you choose.

iii) Write how long you spend with each activity and total up the three columns. The ideal balance is around fifty-six hours on each column.

iv) Now write a list of the names of all the people who really mean something to you. In the same way write down the number of hours that you spend with each during a span of time.

v) Have a good look at your lists and ask yourself the following questions:

Am I pleased with how I spend my time at the moment?

If yes, congratulate yourself and celebrate. If no, would you like to reduce or increase anything?

Would I like to omit something altogether?
Would I like to include something that is not already there?

If so, what?

Am I prepared to let anything go? If so, what?

vi) Taking into account your findings write out the three headings again: Work, Rest and Recreation.

Create your ideal week by writing underneath each heading the activities that you would like to include together with the amount of time to be spent on each.

vii) Do the same with the people that you wish to spend time with.

viii) Is this *really* what you want? If so:

ix) Write out what adjustments need to be made.

x) Am I prepared to make them?

xi) If so, what will I have to do to implement them?

Please identify your first choices and, as far as you can, become aware of what your resulting and inevitable second choices could be.

xii) Am I really prepared to make these changes?

In looking ahead

i) Allow for planning time.

ii) Establish long and short-term projects – one week, month, year, years.

iii) List your priorities.

iv) Block out time for your number one priority.

Remind yourself of your top line priority and keep eliminating lower priorities. Keep asking yourself the question 'Is this really necessary at the moment?' Lower priorities are often easier and keep finding their way to the top of the list.

v) Make requests and ask for help when and where necessary.

vi) Refuse requests when appropriate – eliminate overloading yourself.

vii) Be prepared to delegate – the best way to let go, train and trust others is to do it and learn by doing it.

ix) Be prepared to change course completely – with the awareness of what you are doing and why.

x) Communicate – don't isolate.

xi) Share problems.

Communication

The quality of communication determines the quality of our community at all levels. Good human communication can lead to sharing, harmony, co-operation, love and peace. Failed communication can lead to misunderstanding, selfishness, greed, violence and war. In communicating, collaborating and co-operating well there is a gesture towards a common aim. It fails when the common aim is overlooked or is no longer common.

People can live and work together for a lifetime and continue masquerading behind 'He doesn't talk to me' 'If only you'd said before' 'I never knew' 'Why didn't you say?' It is as though they are living in the same house together and yet with a brick wall around each of them. When one partner leaves the other the reaction could well be 'It's not a bit like him', 'He must be out of his head' or 'He'll soon come to his senses', but the nature of what he has done is very like him and the sadness is that they hardly knew each other.

CO-OPERATION

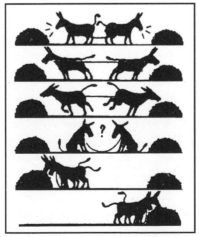

IS BETTER THAN CONFLICT

Practise, practise and keep practising good, open, true communication. Remind yourself of common and individual aims. Invite your partner and friends to practise with you – like an invitation to dance. 'Shall we dance the same dance this evening or shall I continue to dance the tango whilst you continue to dance the waltz?'

'Sing and dance together and be joyous, but let each one of you be alone,
Even as the strings of a lute are alone though they quiver with the same music.'
(Kahlil Gibran, *The Prophet*)

Making requests

Requests are requests – they are not the people who make them. If you make a request which is refused it is the request that is refused – not you. A fear of rejection can lead to not daring to ask. If you find it difficult to ask, start imitating the pattern.

There may be someone that you could start practising making requests with, particularly if it is someone who has difficulty in saying 'no' without feeling awkward. Make a game of it, have fun and practise in small ways to begin with – being genuine and sincere all the time.

Whenever you want to learn a new skill that involves a partner, such as tennis, you need to learn the technique and then practise. Hitting a ball against a brick wall is fine in order to improve your technique but you are still on your own and can usually determine what you are going to get back! Playing tennis with someone else and receiving shots back that you have not necessarily set up increases your scope.

Start to make requests that you are 99.9% sure will be accepted. Then start to make requests that you are 99.9% sure will *not* be accepted, but that, if refused, will not leave you devastated. Get to know what it feels like in a safe way gradually making bigger requests.

- Be straightforward about what you are asking of the other person.
- Make it as brief, clear and simple as possible.
- Be positive in your manner.
- Present yourself and the request expecting the best.
- Believe in it.
- Believe in your worthiness of it.
- Have good intent.
- Omit negatives – 'not' 'no' 'do not' 'sorry' 'awful' 'terrible' and so on.
- Avoid being longwinded – get to the point.

This will show that you appreciate and value yourself and the other person.

- 'I'm awfully sorry but . . .
- 'Would you mind terribly if . . .
- 'I don't know if this is possible but . . .
- 'You're going to hate me for this but could you . . .
- 'I bet you wouldn't do me a favour . . .
- 'I hope you don't mind but . . .

Starting in this way weakens your own position and can be very antagonistic.

Refusing requests

Similarly you can practise saying 'no' in the same way, knowing you are refusing the request and not rejecting the other person.

'The trouble with me is I can't say "no" is often said as a phrase of self appraisal to highlight generosity of spirit. It is also said with real disappointment at just not being able to refuse for fear of not being liked or upsetting the other person.

Saying 'no' at the outset instead of beating around the bush not only helps to prevent you working against your inner self, it also gains respect from others who will know where they stand.

Saying 'yes' too hastily and easily can be like eating up every opportunity to please someone else with little respect for yourself or the other person. Saying 'yes' however could also be the very thing that you require to give you a 'kick start' to open up to new experience. Monitor your habits of saying 'yes' or 'no' and aim to evaluate each request carefully before habitually agreeing or refusing.

You do not have to go through the whole song and dance act of 'I'm awfully sorry but . . . reason/excuse/blame . . . reason/excuse . . .' Simply saying 'no' or 'yes' can be very releasing. Long reasons or excuses can be very tiring. Putting the blame or reason on another person can undermine your own credibility and worth. In not being honest with the other person you are certainly not being honest with yourself and this leads to lack of trust.

No and Yes

These simple words are like closing or opening a gate on a tidal flow. When the gate is open you are welcoming what is coming towards you. When the gate is shut you are keeping it outside yourself. The gate half open and not knowing whether to close it can cause a whirlpool of confusion.

It may not be necessary to accept or refuse the whole thing but just a part of it. A contract in this case can be an agreement between yourself and the other person about what is the other side of the gate – something that has to be worked out together rather than totally accepting or receiving.

Here is a technique that may help you in refusing requests

  i) Visualise yourself in a field which has one gate.

  ii) Do you or do you not want the whole tidal flow of the request as it is at the moment?

  iii) If not, visualise the gate firmly shut. Be clear and convincing in your refusal.

  iv) Can you accept a part of it? If so, which part?

Visualise yourself standing by the gate and be very clear as you state which part you can accept and refuse. Only open the gate to what feels right.

Remember

  Be straightforward and convincing.

  Make the refusal as brief, clear and simple as possible.

LIVERPOOL
JOHN MOORES UNIVERSITY
AVRIL ROBARTS LRC
TEL. 0151 231 4022

Be positive in your manner.

Believe in it.

Omit negatives of 'terribly' 'awfully' and so on.

Avoid being longwinded – get to the point.

Indecision

Indecision, fear and doubt can be the result of not being clear about a situation and may or may not depend upon whether you are in possession of all the facts.

'Be decisive' is the command from outside. 'Either do it or don't do it but make your mind up.' If you are not ready to make a decision the pressure that you may experience can be very destructive. Some suggest that you should make a decision rather than not and if it turns out to be not totally right then make another. Indecision becomes destructive to the point of frustration. Indecision may also be a choice for the fear of losing out on the familiar, however uncomfortable.

However, indecision is not always destructive but the consciousness brought to it determines how you feel about it. *Decide to be indecisive* about a certain issue until you feel ready to do something about it. Truly accept that you have made that decision rather than just worrying about being indecisive which makes it even worse. You can turn what could be destructive into constructive by consciously choosing to delay until you are ready. You can simply say 'I do not know *yet* – I have delayed making a decision.' This will release the tension and can put you in a positive frame of mind and more in control of the situation.

Create a pattern for making decisions. Start in a small way to build your confidence and begin to accept that you are making decisions every day in one way or another. Accept what you are already doing is a direct result of an original decision.

'I decide to go to bed at 11 p.m.' and do it

'I decide to wear red trousers' and do it

'I decide to ask for promotion' and do it

'I decide to communicate with my partner about a difficult issue' and do it

Imitate

Imitate the pattern of making decisions from smaller ones to bigger ones and consciously feel the success of getting into bed at 11 p.m., asking for promotion – and accept the success of it all.

Gradually move from 'being stuck with what is' to creating your own life. It is this creative mode that releases being stuck. A large part of development is stimulated through imitation. Developing the skill of making small decisions creates the pattern for making larger decisions.

Expectations

Through our expectations we can create our own future.

'My father died at fifty six, my mother died at sixty – we don't make old bones in our family.'
'My mother died of cancer, her own mother too and all her brothers and sisters died of cancer. It runs in the family.'

This is programming and this person is expecting to die certainly before the age of seventy and most probably from cancer.

We draw unto ourselves through our expectation. We could expect to be well, to be good enough, to succeed and enjoy high quality life. The happiness of your life depends upon the quality of your thoughts and you can put yourself more in control by expecting what you want.

Affirmations

Most of the day the mind is busy chattering away to itself about this and that – a continuous stream making observations and registering feelings. This inner dialogue forms the current reality and future events based on 'like attracts like'. Every statement that you make is registered and lodged in your 'internal computer'. The mind-chatter cements your experience and *you* become a result of your thinking. Like attracts like just as positive thought patterns create positive living and negative thought patterns creative negative living.

This ceaseless mind-chatter is coloured by past experience and can become very limiting. In relaxation and meditation the mind-chatter appears to be highlighted as you notice your thoughts. It is only when you become aware of this mind-chatter through being still that you begin to realise the kind of world that you are creating for yourself. It is at this point that you can choose to take a positive step to change the current reality and what happens in your future.

An affirmation is a brief powerful statement of something good and positive in the present tense even though it may not be so at the time. It is chosen for its beneficial effect and to change limited experience. The idea is to replace habitual negative thought patterns by feeding the mind positively. Affirmations can be used to relax, energise, comfort, enthuse, inspire, strengthen and so on.

'Every day in every way I am feeling better and better and better' is one of the most famous affirmations created by French physician Emile Coué who encouraged many of his patients back to health through suggesting they repeat this to themselves many times a day and particularly first thing in the morning.

Make up your own affirmations to suit your requirements and in conjunction with your beliefs. You could choose from or adapt any of the following if appropriate. Make sure that you state what you *do* want rather than what you *do not* want. For example 'I do not want this unsatisfactory relationship to continue' binds you to the unsatisfactory relationship. To the contrary 'I deserve a warm loving relationship' is more likely to develop whilst the unsatisfactory relationship dissolves.

The ingredients of a good affirmation are that

IT MUST BE	*YOU MUST*
simple	believe it
clear	believe in your worthiness of it
brief	have good intent
positive	expect it to work
	repeat it regularly

Making decisions is coming easily to me now

Making requests is coming easily to me now: it is the request that is accepted or refused and not me

Refusing requests is coming easily to me now: it is the request that I am refusing and not the person

- I let go all past hurt
- I let go all that is past
- I let go with love
- I forgive . . . for . . .
- I forgive and release myself from . . .
- I am free – you are free
- I am worthy to receive the very best in life
- I am relaxed and happy
- Happiness and wealth are coming to me now
- Vitality and life force are coming to me now
- Energy and power are surging through me now to complete this project in the most effective way
- I accept myself and all my feelings
- Life is wonderful; life is beautiful
- I love myself unconditionally
- I am freely expressing myself creatively and clearly
- I deserve love
- The love of God enfolds me and the power of God flows through me
- Peace is within me; peace is around me
- I let go and let God

You can say your affirmations aloud, quietly to yourself, silently, sing and write them – on your own or with others. A very effective time to repeat them is first thing in the morning and just at the end of your relaxation, meditation and quiet time as the mind is particularly receptive. Make up your own prescription: 'Repeat three times, three times a day, with or without food.' Repeat the statements with belief and expectation. At other times during the day periodically just stop and notice what kind of conservation your mind is having with itself. Notice any negative tendency and become aware of the effect that it could have. Keep checking yourself in this way, making decisions about what you *do* want in your life. Have fun!

Choice

The way that you are is your choice – you have created a life for yourself. The more deeply you examine how you are, what you are, who you are, why you are, when you are and where you are, you will see this to be mostly true. Inevitably there are circumstances over which you appear to have had no control at all – something outside yourself. Of course it depends a lot on how far back you are prepared to look – yesterday, last week, last month, last year, ten years ago, one hundred years or lifetimes ago. Circumstances can become intolerable and your choice of reaction to them continues to formulate the way that you are.

To find yourself in a situation that you do not like may feel as though you are swimming against the tide and as though what you are doing is in direct opposition to what you would like to be doing. Your choice is in the present moment – here and now.

First and second choices

The choice to work all day every day and most evenings means that there is little time for recreation. Having little time for recreation is a direct result of your first choice and there fore becomes your second choice. Other examples of this:

First choice – with limited resources you spend most of your time and money on your home.

Second choice – You have to be very thrifty with clothing, activities, leisure, travel, holidays and socialising.

First choice – You choose to spend most of your time with one person to the exclusion of others.

Second choice – Not seeing your other friends and family may well cause uneasiness.

First choice – You choose to have a 'lie in' on a beautiful sunny morning.

Second choice – You have a late start to the day and miss the sunshine.

First choice – Without unlimited funds you choose not to work.

Second choice – Very little money and maybe lack of mental stimulation.

First choice – You overindulge in food and alcohol.

Second choice – You may put on weight, have a 'thick head' and less money.

The recognition of second choice, however unpleasant, maybe all that is required for you to *change* your first choice or *accept* your second choice.

Are you doing what you want to do?

Stress can be caused by the difference between what you are doing and what your true self needs to be doing – your life desires. You have several choices:

i) You can make changes

ii) You can accept that this is how it must be and accept it graciously. This could involve changing your attitude.

iii) You can choose to neither change or accept and aim to hold the status quo. This is an ideal set up for the 'victim of circumstance' attitude of 'Why me?' and the martyr syndrome.

These are all choices although some are more obvious than others. Time comes to ask yourself – 'What am I doing?' When you do this and come up with an answer then ask yourself 'Why is that?' and when you have found an answer ask yourself again 'Why is that?' and repeat this several times until you reach the revealing truth. This is a simple and valuable technique.

Conscious choice

Begin to make conscious choices of how you would like to be and really mean it. *You really do have a choice in forming your future.*

Basic requirements of conscious choice

Choose to be positive, in the here and now, with good intent.

i) Accentuate the positive and eliminate the negative. For example 'I choose not to be late for meetings' gives emphasis to the lateness without giving an alternative. The words 'not' 'never' 'no' emphasise the negative and should not appear in conscious choice. 'I choose to be on time for meetings' gives emphasis to being on time with an alternative.

ii) The moment of 'now' is the most powerful. It is the point for change. You can remind yourself by saying 'This is the first day of the rest of my life'.

iii) Having love and respect for yourself and others will lead you to choices that are in your own best interest and in the best interest for others around you.

You can consciously choose to create how you want to be and the following is a practical suggestion of how to do that. It is not necessary to write it down but its strength is in its simplicity and writing can help to cement that.

Exercise

You need a notepad to be kept just for this purpose, entitled 'Choices'.

i) Create a picture in your mind of how you would like things to be *now*, at the present moment, rather than how you do not want them to be or concerning yourself about the future. This may involve any or all areas of your life – physical wellbeing, personal relationships, mental attitude, feelings and spirituality. For example, you may picture yourself as slim, healthy, enjoying your life without cigarettes, experiencing a wonderful relationship and an immensely satisfying job. Imagine *every* aspect of your life in detail.

ii) Now refer to your notepad, opening up onto a double page and start to create how you would like things to be *now* on paper. You may like to write it out, use symbols, paint or draw.

iii) With attention to the basic requirements of conscious choice as outlined above begin to verbalise just one basic choice which will help bring this situation about in a clear and concise way. Start your statement: 'I (your first name) choose to . . .' Use the back of your notepad and write it out. Take time to get it just right. Play around with it until it feels strong. Make two more choices in the same way to support your description and picture of how you would like your life to be at the moment. 'I (your first name) choose to . . .' 'I (your first name) choose to . . .' Now you can have three clear, concise statements that you can easily recall and that have already begun to make an impact. Repeat them over and over again until you begin to feel them in your bones. Refer to the front of your pad and write them out.

Prescription

Now write them out as a prescription in the following way:

Date . . . .

i) I choose to . . .

ii) I choose to . . .

iii) I choose to . . .

Each choice to be repeated three times, four times a day, with the book:

on waking in the morning

mid morning

mid afternoon

at bedtime.

To be reviewed in a month.

As you look at your book say the three choices out loud. The first choice three times, the second choice three times and the third choice three times. Really believe it and allow time to digest. In this way you will be consciously choosing how you want your life to be by repeating each statement twelve time a day. Soon you will begin to feel these choices working in your life. Realise and fully accept that you have created a pattern for change and believe in the power of this most simple technique.

What *was probable*
Is *now possible*
And is *definitely preferable*

As you notice changes write them out in your book under the headings Developing/ Dissolving.

Review each prescription every month and prepare to make new choices to replace the others that you have already set in motion. Only repeat the prescription if it still feels absolutely right to do so.

Three choices repeated three times, four times a day, is a perfect prescription for you to take charge of your life. For example:

i) 'I choose to look after myself and improve my physical wellbeing'.

It will now be far more natural to eat well, breathe well, take exercise, express your emotions, practise relaxation and have adequate rest and sleep. If you find yourself slipping back recognise your first and second choice. Repeat the statement to yourself if you wish – it is your choice. Change it if you need in order to make it more effective. If you go to light up another cigarette, make yet another cup of coffee, pour yet another drink, stay huddled up in front of the television for hours on end, zoom to the fridge for another chocolate – say to yourself 'I . . . choose to look after myself and improve my physical wellbeing.'

ii) 'I . . . choose to communicate clearly and in truth with my family and friends.' Remind yourself of this when you start to fly off the handle and/or avoid confrontation. Let the positive choice seep into your system and work for you.

Sure, you will catch yourself out at times but avoid giving yourself a hard time for there are no success or fail marks and no intention of giving anything up. Just develop and dissolve. The power of it all is in its simplicity. Choose from small things to bigger more meaningful things.

The following are a few suggestions that you may like to sue as a pattern but it is essential that you make your own positive choices that feel right for you.

'I . . . choose to look after myself and improve my physical wellbeing'

'I . . . choose to express my feelings'

'I . . . choose to enjoy warm loving relationships'

'I . . . choose to have a quiet time to myself once a day'

'I . . . choose to be kind and true to myself'

'I . . . choose to live and love my life today'

'I . . . choose to go running every morning'.

Fourfold remedy

Old habits which you no longer require become obsolete – they have served their purpose and have had their time. Forget about spending a lot of time and energy in stopping old habits. Begin to develop new habits through conscious choice and allow the obsolete ways to fade into the background. There is a cosmic law –

'That which is nourished grows
that which is not nourished dies'

Increasingly there are links being made between illness and disease and anger, fear, grief and resentment. Every thought affects the body in some way and the ancient teaching of Patanjali suggests a delightful fourfold remedy to develop the 'undisturbed calmness of mind' by cultivating:

- friendliness toward the happy
- compassion for the unhappy
- delight in the virtuous
- indifference toward the wicked

In developing these attitudes the mind becomes more clear, calm and peaceful however busy you are and the qualities of the heart are developed. These positive attitudes are very conducive to good health and wellbeing.

5 Help Yourself to Health

Physical and mental attitudes

Longevity is only any good if it allows you to enjoy the quality of your life. Lifespan may well be increased through careful attention to the physical body but it is your attitude that will make it worthwhile. A good aim is to die young as late as you can.

You can raise your tolerance level to stress by really looking after yourself and attending to the well-being of your body, mind, emotions and spirit – recognising that each affects the other and is an integral part of the whole. Build up your reserves of strength by the way that you live life – and live it well. You can change and enhance every cell in your body.

Look after yourself

Eat well, breathe well, exercise well and learn to relax.

Occupation, leisure and recreation

Your occupation is the way in which you occupy your time. Wherever you are bored, tired and lazy is where you invest least energy and have least interest. Wherever you have most excitement, frustration, tension and anger is where you invest most energy and have most interest. This may sound obvious but when you examine how you are at home, with your partner, friends and in your main occupation you may be quite surprised at the outcome. The investment of energy is in direct relationship to the interest.

Your attitude to the way in which you use your leisure time can make it into hard graft, a labourious chore or a pleasant pastime. To bring the attitude of 'work', 'deadlines', and 'competing' into leisure is not ceasing or changing but just continuing and repeating the already overloaded system in the same way.

Include a non-competitive hobby or pastime which will give you the opportunity to involve and devote yourself completely without the external pressure of 'matching up to' or 'being better than'. Being 'lost' in the object of your attention is a most releasing, refreshing and re-creative process.

Strong physical exercise can complement hours spent over a typewriter just as stimulating conversation and debate can complement tiring physical work. After a day spent 'in your head' when the thinking process has been taxed, then rolling up your sleeves and doing the dishes, scrubbing the kitchen floor, digging the garden or cleaning the car can be very welcome activities that require little thought – mindless activity. If you spend a lot of time alone you may find that the brushing of shoulders in the hustle and bustle of the marketplace is just what you need to shift the inward attitude.

In his delightful little book *Workers of the world – unite, and stop working* Jim Haynes suggests the creation of the verb 'to fuller' in honour of Buckminster Fuller who, he says, 'epitomizes joyful energy spending' and had already written a book himself entitled *I seem to be a verb*. Loving your work and job satisfaction are high on the list after love and good relationships. Aim to give meaning to your life through your work and meaning to your work through your life.

Fresh air and sunshine

If your main occupation is indoors be very strict with yourself and put the priority of having a break in the fresh air high on your list. This can have an exhilarating effect and you will return to work refreshed. If possible have at least fifteen minutes of sunshine a day as it is a valuable source of vitamin D. When sunbathing respect the power of the sun's burning rays.

Smoking, alcohol, tranquillisers

These can help and hinder. Take responsibility for what is right for you. An overindulgence in any or all of these three may have a disastrous effect upon your health. If you have cause for concern about tranquillisers please refer to the appendix.

Touch

The quality of bonding, holding, rocking and stroking that you experienced as a tiny baby being born and a young child has an effect upon you for the rest of your life. If it was sadly lacking at that time there may be a resultant craving for it or repulsion of it. The sense of touch is something that can feed you emotionally – it can comfort, excite, soothe and stimulate. It can be a source of caring and feeling cared for. When someone becomes accustomed to physical contact with another person – partner, parent, child, or friend it becomes part of their emotional food. If at any time it is suddenly no longer available, maybe due to separation, divorce or death, then that person can be left bereft, distraught and with a very real feeling of emotional starvation that can lead to becoming 'touch-hungry'.

Western culture tends to be 'touch-shy' which is unfortunate because the touch of another human being is the source of great and deep comfort and is a basic human need which, if ignored, can lead to a feeling of isolation and deprivation. It has been noted that some people who have high blood pressure can reduce their blood pressure from the comfort of stroking a beloved pet regularly every day and being closely in tune with another restful heart beat.

Giving and receiving a massage is not only a source of deep comfort, it can improve communication, enhance relationships and can be a deeply healing experience. Don't wait until you get something wrong with you before you have a massage. Realise the value of it whilst you are well. You can learn how to massage from courses and books and then practise on a loved one or seek out a friend who is willing to be a guinea pig.

Smile

Develop the smiling habit and include at least three other people during the day that you would not normally smile at. You will be amazed at the positive effect that this can have for yourself and others. Mother Theresa says 'Peace starts with a smile' – why not put it to the test?

Other people

Actively seek out the company of other people whose presence you enjoy either because you find them interesting, stimulating, uplifting, comforting, funny, loving or for any other reason. Being with people with whom you have little rapport or who bore you out of your mind may be a reflection on both parties. This can be draining and depleting or an area that can lead to growth and understanding. Remind yourself why you are there in that situation with those people before you hastily change or move. Do remember that every thought affects the body in some way.

Fun, laughter and a sense of humour

> '*A merry heart doeth good like a medicine*'
>
> **(Proverbs 17 : 22.)**

Seriousness can damage your health. Laughter and a sense of humour have a profound effect upon the body and mind. A sense of humour enables you to release a lot of suppressed thought, hence the success of comedians and comedy at the theatre. People laugh sometimes in an uncontrollable way in desperate situations in order to release the tension. In his book *Anatomy of an Illness* Norman Cousins tells how he used his sense of humour as a vital and contributory factor to his recovery from a crippling illness. In writing about creativity and longevity he refers to two brilliant men – Pablo Casals and Albert Schweitzer. 'Albert Schweitzer always believed that the best medicine for any illness he might have was the knowledge that he had a job to do, plus a good sense of humour. He once said that the disease tended to leave him rather rapidly because it found so little hospitality inside his body.' He would include a humorous tale every evening at dinner to help raise the spirits of the young doctors and nurses in the Schweitzer hospital.

Laughter reaches the body through the soul and has a most positive effect upon the lungs and intestines so improving the breathing, digestion and elimination. This is known as internal jogging. Norman Cousins reported how his blood sedimentation rate lowered due to laughter and was consequently responsible for the continuing reduction of inflammation around his joints.

Make sure that you have some fun in your life – something that lifts and brings good hearted amusement. If you have at least one good laugh every day you are well blessed – something that makes you and others laugh. If you have difficulty in finding something to laugh about then laugh at yourself – you are *bound* to find something.

Treat

Give yourself a treat at least once a day. Make it something that you would not normally do – use your imagination and have fun. Have a warm luxurious bath with perfumed oils; eat a juicy pear or orange in the bath; sensuously stretch across the carpet and then curl up with a teddy bear for five minutes; run down a hill singing, laughing, shouting or yelling; day dream; watch the sun rise and set. Make up your own. Everyone has time for a treat for it can be as brief as you wish. Adopt the attitude that it is something really special and just for you. Develop the treat time to include an extra one each week, month and year and set out to enjoy it to the full.

Loneliness

The impression of loneliness can be a comparison between when you were not alone and your experience of aloneness now. Loneliness can repel for like attracts like. There are ways of shifting attitude to loneliness. When you say to yourself 'I am *so* lonely' you are affirming that this is so. Play a game with words and change one letter in the word so that instead you say to yourself 'I am so *lovely*'. Loveliness attracts loveliness. If you say this to yourself often enough as an affirmation you can begin to *feel* lovely, as indeed you are. If you say to yourself as you walk through town 'I am so lovely' you may be quite surprised how your whole aura changes to attract other people to you. Your face, physical bearing and whole demeanour will be a point of attraction instead of rejection and loneliness.

Looking at the word in another way – 'alone' when broken into two becomes 'all one'. The word 'all' refers to the whole amount. It is used as a prefix to many other words. All seeing, All knowing etc. The word 'one' refers to unity, united, the same and unchanging. A feeling of being All One is quite different from being alone – try it. 'I am All One – an integral part of the whole and as such cannot be alone' – solitary maybe but never alone.

Bless the loneliness that can become All One and lovely. Being alone is a state of separation. Being All One is being at one and attuned to that which is united and unchanging.

This is not suggesting a remedy for loneliness but another attitude to bring to it.

Gratitude

Several years ago a lady came to see me in a very sad and distressed state. She talked and talked. After quite a long time the conversation slowly turned from complaints and criticism to appreciation and gratitude. I asked her if she might like to continue in that vein and write down all the things that she could be thankful for in some way, however small, and telephone me the next day to let me know how she got on. Hesitantly she agreed to start writing a list when she got into bed that night. It was a vastly different tone of voice that I heard when she rang early the following morning with the news that she had filled nearly four large sheets of paper, fallen asleep and continued to write when she awoke in the morning. This had become a source of great interest and comfort to her. Although her unhappy situation had not changed *she* had *changed towards it* and had been able to 'lift' herself up out of it as she dwelt upon the good things in her life.

She had started with her list with seemingly minor things like 'I am in a warm bed with a hot water bottle. I have a cup of tea. I can see my bedroom light. I can hear the traffic outside. I have a good washing machine' and began to expand to ' I love my little cat and she loves me too. I can walk to the beach, pick up shells and stones and smell the sea air every day. I can walk to the shops and buy my own food' and later in the list 'I am thankful for trees, the sea, the sun, the air, the moors, Sundays, Mondays, Tuesdays and all the other days in the week' and so on. She had begun to look outside herself again.

Part of the dictionary definition of gratitude is 'an inclination to return kindness'. Use this most simple and valuable exercise in your own life not only when things are going well but when they are not going well too.

Emotional expression

Fear is the greatest barrier to expressing our feelings. Emotions are not separate from the mind or the body – they are all affected by each other. Feelings that are associated with the heart centre have many expressions to support that, for the heart can ache, sing, sink, miss a beat, spill over, break, turn over, bleed, cry, soar, melt and so on. The body has an intelligence of its own and reflects most beautifully what is happening in the mind and emotions.

The 'stiff upper lip' desperate to hold something back can produce internal acidity, bitterness, caustic speech and criticism, eating into your gut or 'eating your heart out'. Desperate to hold something back we parade and dance behind our own masks, forgetting almost who we are, frightened to confront ourselves let alone anyone else. Building emotional fences and brick walls are all very efficient ways of keeping something in, out or back. It takes a lot of effort and energy to suppress feelings and the more energy it takes, the more frightening is the thought of the new powerfulness of these emotions if we should let them go.

Dare to share your feelings – first of all fully accepting them yourself. Really own your feelings however wonderful, devastating, bewildering or horrific they appear to be. Accept them as a part of you and part of the whole. Laugh with them and cry with them. When you feel more comfortable with them start to practise sharing them where it is safe and appropriate; that is, with the right person whether nearest and dearest, friend or a stranger in the form of a trained counsellor. It is at these times that we could all do with friends who have huge shoulders to cry on and massive ears to listen.

Practise in small ways first of all when you feel frightened, upset, angry, overjoyed, bewildered or whatever. Let it out in direct ways with the person concerned where and when you can. Begin to let down the barriers with care so that you can have respect for yourself and others as you decently expose yourself. Being vulnerable is daring to feel and live and to give opportunity to the joy and sorrow that lies deep within your being, having respect for that within yourself and within others.

Grief

Expressing our grief is a natural and healthy process. Not recognising, not accepting and trying to hide and suppress grief can be most unhealthy and lead to much confusion, distress and illness. Termination of pregnancy, miscarriage, still birth, death of a beloved, friend, animal, figurehead, empire, marriage, business, community and so on all require a period of mourning and grief.

'The grief has to be in the background because I feel so awful' was a statement made by an elderly lady who, within a period of two years, had lost her husband, best friend, daughter, had a colostomy and moved from a house that she had loved and lived in for forty years. The 'awfulness' was part of the grief and accepting that brought an enormous sense of relief. It brought the grief to the foreground with full recognition of the present moment. Taking heavy medication of sleeping pills and tranquillisers was an attempt to *mask* the feeling and to get through the most traumatic stage but being physically sick was an attempt by the body to express the feeling of grief.

If grief has been held back in the past it will still seek an outlet. You may have experienced separation, divorce, bereavement, or children leaving home, and been able to cope reasonably well and then, all of a sudden, when you change your job, or home or your dearest pet dies, you can find yourself experiencing an extraordinary, seemingly inappropriately traumatic, reaction to the loss – quite out of proportion. The suppressed grief from the past has begun to find an outlet.

> 'The grief that does not speak, whispers across the o'er fraught heart and bids it break'.
> (Shakespeare *Macbeth*)

The first stage of grief can take the form of shock, disorientation, numbness, disbelief, pretending nothing has happened and hiding or covering it up.

The second stage is the dawn of realisation of the truth that can manifest in blaming oneself or others, being very angry and resentful, feeling dreadful in every way, manifesting similar symptoms of illness as the deceased, crying, withdrawing and loss of interest in life. This is a healthy stage of grief.

The third stage is to have a genuine sense of recovery and acceptance having *allowed yourself to feel*. This is the stage of true adjustment and getting used to living and being without.

Let the four seasons come and go and let them carry the grief too. Resisting, refusing, getting stuck in the past are all holding on with a refusal to let go.

Lose or let go

There is a distinct difference between these two very similar words. To *lose* or to *loose* – that is the question.

To lose (dict.) is to be deprived of. This is where you are deprived of someone or something – by someone or something and you are not in control of losing. 'I have lost my beloved – my beloved has been taken from me.'

To loose (dict.) is to release from bonds, to detach, to set free, to undo. This is to consciously let go and you are in control of the loosening. 'I have loosened my beloved. I have set free, let go, released my beloved.'

These two attitudes take on very different meanings. 'Losing' to 'loosening' is simple and yet can be most difficult. It is the difference between holding onto and letting go. Letting go can be most rewarding, releasing, expansive and wonderful.

Ethnic cultures sing and dance about everything in their lives – birth, maturity, work, play, praise, pain, joy, sorrow, sickness, war, peace, thanksgiving, harvest, loss, death and so on. Death is honoured and recognised for what it is – a passage and passing through to another dimension.

Western civilisation has tended to underrate the value of creative expression as part of everyday life and health. Giving expression to activity is one of the healthiest pursuits. Theatre and the arts play a cathartic role and have been recognised as such since the early days of ancient Greek tragedy. The creative therapies of drama, art, music and play have a most subtle and profound way of leading the imagination to heal and to give expression to emotion that lies dormant or suppressed.

In the same way it is sometimes more acceptable to us to feel the sadness and pain of other people's losses than our own and resonate and identify with others. Soap opera, film, theatre, music, poetry, art, sculptor and nature all present us with an opportunity to identify and release that which we are holding within us and cry with delight, joy and sadness.

Helping others

Wanting to help others is a constructive way of working with your own joy and sorrow. Love, understanding, listening, laughing, crying together and helping in practical ways are the best medicine in the world. In helping others you are helping yourself.

In the late 19th century medical papers were written to support the link between suppressed emotion and cancer and yet it is still not widely accepted. With our 'stiff upper lips' and 'bleeding hearts' we are prime targets. We set ourselves up for it as we set our own stage for the illness to play a leading role in our lives and to express physically what we are unable to do mentally and emotionally. It is choice made at a most fundamental level and not to be denied. The body is no fool.

Suppressing and denying feelings takes an enormous amount of strength and saps valuable creativity. Developing a natural creative talent can begin to channel that energy. Everyone has their own unique talent or talents to express and their own 'song to sing'. Big mistakes are made when you try to sing someone else's song and deny the value of your own. Some

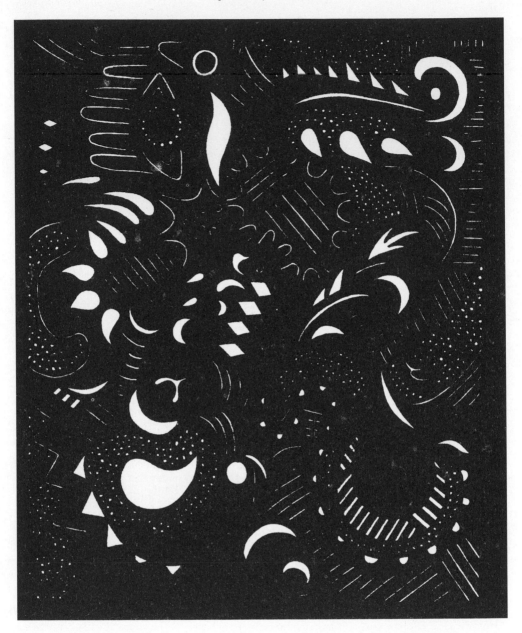

people live all their lives trying to be good at something because someone else is and still feel unfulfilled even though they may become proficient at another's talent.

Freedom in expression

Not long ago a young woman came to practise Yoga and meditation in a class at our local college. She asked if she could see me on her own to discuss some difficulties that she was having. Behind this beautiful smiling friendly face hid the deep sadness and hurt in her eyes and heart. She talked, I listened. I talked, she listened – and so on. This was quite different from 'we talked'. I asked her what she *really loved doing*. 'This might sound really silly' she said, 'but I love doodling.' I asked her if she felt like sharing her doodles with me and she agreed. Weeks, months, and many doodles have gone by since that first meeting and Kim tells you in her own words:

'Thinking back to my childhood I remember quite vividly if I was ever at a loose end, feeling nervous, afraid, shy or whatever – I would soon pick up a material of some sort, be it grass, leaves, sand or ink and start creating various shapes into patterns – the patterns of my mind.

As far back as I can remember my mind always seemed muddled with a bombardment of thoughts, bouncing from one side of my head to the other and the more I questioned them the more out of control my head became. Through my doodling I found a tunnel for the turmoil of confusion to disperse, so leaving my mind clearer and my body more relaxed.

During my late teens, early twenties I suffered various mental disturbances and through my doodling and counselling I found it possible to come to terms with my problems and accept them, leaving my mind free and light from the heavy burdens of the past.

When I feel uptight and out of control I sit with a blank piece of paper and attack it with all my fears, worries etc. Each shape I draw represents a different emotion and as I draw each circle or line I shed away a little more of the tension that has built up inside me. When I have finished the picture I feel more relaxed. I can now look at the problem in a different light as I have separated it from myself. It is as though it belongs to another person. I'm not saying that when I feel depressed and overrun with problems I sit down and draw them all away but I am able to separate them from myself for long enough to put them into their proper perspective and deal with them in a positive way.'

Kim Faulkner

Singing your own song

This moving example of emotional expression is an inspiration. For sure, this lovely girl has been 'singing her own song' and as a result has been asked by many people to frame her doodles and share them even further.

There are times when certain situations seem insurmountable and even the imagination enlarges upon it for you. Talk about it, sing about it, dance, play a musical instrument, write about it, draw, paint or shape it with clay. Develop your own craft and way of giving expression to your feelings. It is not necessary to be a great writer, musician, artist, painter or potter in the accepted way but with a creativity that is yours and yours alone. Just *be yourself* and use what is appropriate to you as a way of getting it outside yourself rather than within. If you choose to write then write and keep writing. What you choose to do with it is totally up to you. Maybe the very writing is sufficient in itself or you may choose to share it with someone else – post it as a letter, read it, ask a friend to read it or even bury it, burn it or drown it if you feel it has served its purpose. The very ritual of burying, burning or drowning can be letting it go just as we let one another go at the end of physical life. You may find that you have tapped into your own creativity which was longing for expression. Sharing it with other people is an invitation for them to do the same.

The finest orchestra and choir are a collection of people with their own talents in expression and not a collection of people who are perfect singers and musicians. Hold on to your dreams and express that which is within you however openly or privately. Give power to your life in expression and let your dream and creativity become a challenge and channel and a hope for the future. Graciously accept and value the depth of your being, and in the stillness, when you know that your life is truly in expression, you are 'singing your own song' and 'in tune' with life itself.

6 The Breath as a Key

Breathing is the constant change between having air inside and outside the body. Air enters the body in one form and leaves in another – an exchange of what is needed and what is not needed. Respiration is a natural automatic function and is intimately linked to all other body functions. If you had to organise your breathing for the day you certainly would not survive very long.

The breathing rate and pattern is like a barometer of mental and emotional states. When you are excited the breathing rate increases dramatically and when quiet, calm and rested the breathing rate lowers. However, the breath is also something that can be consciously affected and controlled for specific purposes and *you can change your mental and emotional state by the way in which you breathe*.

Life-force

There is a quality in the air known as life-force. It exists in the air and the air exists in it. It penetrates the whole body even where air cannot reach. In Yoga this is known as prana – present in all living matter and the elements – the light and warmth of the sun, wind in the trees, food that we eat, water that we drink.

This same life-force is available to every living creature and we can consciously draw upon it. Where there is breath there is life-force. Where there is breath there is opportunity to increase the life-force, if the spirit is willing, and any increase enhances vitality and well-being. Life-force is an electrical potential. Vitality and health can be seen as an expression of abundant electrical charge by ion exchange, tension, electrical potential and harmony of all physical systems.

Ions

Electrical charges in the atmosphere are called ions and they affect all living things electro-magnetically. Ions are electrically charged particles into which atoms or molecules of certain chemicals are disassociated by solution in water and which make such solution a conductor of electricity. Ions are present in the air that we breathe in a ratio of negative and positive concentration.

Negative ions include oxygen and nitrogen. They form the atmospheric life-force and are to be found in abundance from the sun, in the countryside, mountains, hills, by masses of water in movement or in the course of evaporation, rivers, fountains and showers. Negative ions have a beneficial effect encouraging mental and physical vitality as the respiration slows down and blood pressure lowers.

Positive ions include carbon dioxide and are found in abundance in crowded towns, cities and buildings. They have a detrimental effect resulting in depletion, mental and physical inertia, poor respiration, anxiety and aggression. Dust, fumes, fog and smoke trap and absorb the negative ions rendering them neutral.

Environment

In any given place there is an ideal balance between the soil, climate, vegetation, plant, animal and human life. As one part changes the balance is disturbed creating a need for change within the other component parts. It is not wise to disturb the balance too often. Human beings are just part of the environment. When the environment or anything else in it changes it is necessary to adapt in order to maintain a semblance of balance.

If there is a disturbance in the environment – wait and watch very carefully and be prepared to adapt in whatever way may be necessary. It is not good any longer relying on past rules, regulations and patterns to guide us as they are fast becoming outmoded and obsolete. Now, like never before we have to do our best to keep up with the times – whatever that may mean in any particular circumstance.

From above we are showered with a highly charged life-force in the atmosphere from the sun and air. From below the earth absorbs and stores this wonderful life-force. In between, the human organism undergoes incessant exchange with the play of cosmic and terrestrial energy. Lungs and skin are our exchange surfaces like real electrical sponges. All the surfaces of the body, right down to the walls of the cells within the body, have differing energy potential. We are a vast bio-electrical system with energy continually passing through us. With too little we become tired and lifeless; with too much or incorrect use we become over-excited and neurotic. We must learn how to absorb the energy and use it in the best way possible. In becoming aware of areas that are charged in different ways we can create change within ourselves by simply being in those areas. Although these areas may be quite different they can also live quite close to each other and you can pass from one to another within short distances.

Highly charged areas are very invigorating – places where nothing stops the wind and conifers grow in abundance.

Moderately charged areas are more sheltered with valleys, deep bays by the sea, woods, forests, pastures and vegetation.

Lowly charged areas have a calming effect on nervous people and include deep valleys, under-growth, 'deep cut-rivers', abundant vegetation, climbing plants and ferns.

'Zilch' charged areas are where man has polluted the atmosphere in industrial areas and overcrowded concrete jungles. These are places that literally draw the energy out of the body. Trees, gardens, parks, streams, rivers, water fountains all play a major part in the balance of the atmosphere in town planning. The wildlife that abounds along the railway embankments not only adds charm but gives very definite benefits to crowded city life.

In addition to becoming aware of these areas we can also avoid insulating ourselves too much behind closed doors, concrete, windows and metal with plastic furniture and wall coverings, nylon carpets and synthetic clothing, which neutralises free life-force.

Life absorbing organs

Skin

The skin absorbs life-force from the air and sun. When possible let your skin breathe those life-giving rays and not just to acquire a tan. Whenever possible wear natural fibres of wool, cotton, silk and wear leather shoes.

Tongue

The tongue extracts life-force from food and drink. If food still has flavour in it then it still has life-force and it should be chewed until the flavour has finally gone in order to absorb the maximum life-force from it. Notice, in particular, when you are in need of refreshment, how, as soon as you drink or eat something, you feel refreshed. There is no way that digestion has taken place in that moment of swallowing. It is the absorbing qualities of the tongue that have given the feeling of stimulation.

Nerve endings in nasal cavities

Air is the main nutrient without which we would not exist for very long. Breathing through the nose conditions the air – warms, moistens and frees it from dust as the hairs inside the nose do a grand sweeping job. Air stimulates the delicate nerve endings in the nasal cavities. These nerve endings are linked with the vital nerve centres in the body. Therefore breathing through the nose can have a direct effect upon the level of arousal. Dilating the nostrils stimulates the intake of air and gives signals to the whole respiratory system so that maximum life-force is absorbed.

The more subtle qualities of smell are also detected by breathing through the nose. The nerve endings which contact the olfactory region of the brain are stimulated. Smell has a very definite effect upon the whole psyche.

Air cells in the lungs – alveoli

There are over six hundred million sacs in the lungs and these allow the exchange and passage of life-force, oxygen and waste materials across their surfaces and to the blood. The efficiency of this depends a lot upon the condition of lungs and the quality of the blood.

Breathing action

Oxygen is required to burn up waste matter and purify the blood stream. At the inhalation only the required amount of oxygen is absorbed by the lungs and at the exhalation only a small amount of total carbon dioxide is breathed out. During exercise the circulation demands more oxygen and so the lungs draw in and release as required. There are two main sets of muscles used for breathing – those which move the chest and those that form the diaphragm which separates the chest from the abdomen.

The diaphragm

This is a horizontal dome-shaped muscular sheet forming a ceiling for the abdomen, which contains stomach and intestines, and a floor for the chest, which contains heart and lungs. There are sheets of muscle in between the ribs and these are at work during quiet natural breathing. There are other chest muscles which, when developed, together with the sheets of muscles between the ribs, increase the capacity of the lungs and are usually well developed in athletes and where there is an intention to increase the expanded chest and capacity of the lungs, for example, opera singers and weight lifters. The natural healthy way of breathing involves using all parts of the lungs, that is the lower lobes as well as the middle and top.

It is worth watching a cat, dog or baby sleeping and notice the way in which they breathe. Notice the inhalation – the rib cage expands and the abdomen slightly swells as the air rushes into the lungs; there is a slight pause and then the exhalation. The same mechanism contracts as the air rushes out of the lungs – then a slight pause, and so on. This should be natural to us too but somehow we seem to have lost the natural and gentle art of breathing correctly in a relaxed manner.

If short of breath the natural tendency is to breathe in deeply into the chest but this is only part of the picture. There is far more available if the diaphragm is used in an intelligent way. There is no advantage in trying too hard to breathe in deeply and forcing the lungs as this can actually work against the person with bronchitis, asthma, panic attacks, erratic breathing and shortness of breath.

> 'The mind may also be calmed by expulsion and retention of the breath'
>
> (How to Know God, *Patanjali I v34*.)

Expulsion of the breath

The key in the expulsion is the letting go, the releasing and relaxing. One of the greatest gifts that we can allow ourselves is to let go physically, mentally and emotionally. In being attached to material possessions, wealth, people and pleasurable experience we can become imprisoned by them. Physical and mental stress and tension are often a result of holding on tight and not letting go. We can *use* the exhalation to let go physically, mentally and emotionally.

Retention of the breath

During the retention of the breath out and in there is a subtle opportunity of stillness, where the mind can become still and unruffled. Often in absolute absorption in the object of concentration the breath stops. You might like to check that for yourself some time. It is as though you simply forget to breathe for a while – the mind is so still. This is the stillness that the harassed mind pursues. Sometimes it happens by chance but we can also elicit this stillness. It is available at any time if we care and choose to contact it.

Hyperventilation

During times of stress the breathing automatically becomes rapid and shallow, only using about one tenth of the total lung capacity. This prepares the body for fight-or-flight and is ideal for that stage. However, it is not necessary to continue that way of breathing after the immediate 'action-stations'. There is a tendency in today's 'hurry sickness' world to remain in that state – anxious and pressed for time. With short shallow breaths there is a tendency to rid the lungs of too much carbon dioxide which is required to keep the acid-alkaline levels of the blood in balance. Overbreathing can be the result of this state and it is a common symptom of incorrect breathing. The effects can include dizziness, headaches, cramps, nervousness, phobias, shortness of breath, muscle tremors, tingling feet and hands, chest pain, a feeling of unreality, excessive exhaustion, fatigue and indigestion.

If this applies to you please also refer to the Appendix entitled *Anxiety attack, panic and hyperventilation.*

Whereas deep steady breathing can induce calmness, irregular, rapid, shallow, uncontrolled breathing can trigger and bring about despondency and mental disturbance.

In order to combat tension the first thing to do is to slow down the rhythm of the breath to approximately five to six breaths per minute and then regulate the rhythm of each cycle so that inhalation and exhalation are even.

How to restore correct breathing

Many people have lost the art of breathing properly. Restoration of correct breathing is an essential part of re-establishing a more calm and relaxed frame of mind. It is necessary therefore to develop the movement of the diaphragm and reduce the attention on having a large expanded chest which in itself can be the cause of tension in the upper back, neck and shoulders. What needs to happen is the *gentle coaxing of allowing air to enter the lungs* and to *leave without force*. This can be done by getting to know your diaphragm through the Complete Diaphragm Breath but before doing so it is advisable to learn to relax.

Breathing exercises

The aim of these techniques is to quieten the mind, balance the whole system and become aware of the expansion of the life-force. They are now widely used in clinics, health centres and hospitals for the restoration of good breathing patterns as preventive medicine and to aid recovery after coronary heart failure, reduce high blood pressure, ease anxiety, help with the reduction of tranquillisers, sleep problems and so on.

It may seem strange to suggest the restoration of a good breathing pattern to someone who has been breathing all their lives and may be sixty or seventy years old. However, when understood and practised it becomes obvious to some that they have been breathing incorrectly for most of their lives. The re-establishment of natural good breathing patterns can offer a new lease on life.

The following exercises are a suggestion to:

- re-establish a healthy way of breathing to maximise the efficiency of the lungs
- to clear the nostrils and sinus cavities
- to balance the nervous system, release tension, encourage control over the breath and therefore over the mind and emotions
- to become aware of the breath and expand the life-force
- to increase powers of concentration
- to calm down.

The best time to practise is first thing before breakfast, after physical exercises and during periods of natural break throughout the day or evening. Never practise immediately after eating as the body will be more concerned with digestion. Always have a clean handkerchief with you before you start.

Clear the nostrils

Take up the *Basic Sitting Position* as referred to in the appendix (page 142) and prepare to clear the nostrils by first blowing your nose well – one nostril at a time.

i) Close the right nostril with the right thumb and blow out of the left nostril quite strongly four or five times. Then breathe in and out once or twice very gently and evenly through that nostril.

ii) Repeat on the other side. Close the left nostril with the ring finger on the right hand and blow out of the right nostril four or five times. Then breathe in and out gently and evenly through that same nostril just once or twice.

iii) Release the hand and breathe naturally and evenly through both nostrils.

i *The Complete Diaphragm Breath*

The aim of this breath is to draw the maximum amount of air into all parts of your lungs and especially to activate the lower lobes through *gentle encouragement* rather than forcing or trying too hard.

i) Lie flat in the *basic lying down position* (see Appendix.)

ii) Release any tight clothing particularly around the neck, chest, waist. Throughout this exercise please keep the movement in the diaphragm and abdomen and the mid- and upper-chest area quite still.

iii) Relax from the top of your head down to the tips of your toes.

iv) Place the palm of your left hand over your navel and your right hand on your upper chest near the throat.

v) Thoroughly exhale and draw the abdomen in so that the left hand sinks in. Throughout the whole exercise the mid and upper chest, throat and right hand remain still.

vi) *As you begin to inhale allow your diaphragm to lower and your abdomen to slightly swell, pushing against your left hand (Figure i) (mid and upper chest, throat and right hand quite still).

vii) Hold the breath for a moment, becoming aware of the expansion in the lungs particularly low down and sideways and, when the natural impulse comes to release the breath, then

viii) Begin to draw the abdomen in as you slowly exhale from the base of the lungs first, then left hand sinking, the right hand staying quite still and the diaphragm resumes its first position (as in Figure ii).

ix) When the natural impulse comes to breathe in again do so and repeat this wave-like motion from vi)* several times without straining until it begins to feel natural, comfortable and very relaxing.

Notice how the air is *pulled in* and *flows out* by the controlling action of the diaphragm. Now roll over so that you are lying prone and just rest with your head on one side. Notice your breath and let it become quite natural. Rest and relax completely and concentrate on the expansion in the sides and back of the lungs.

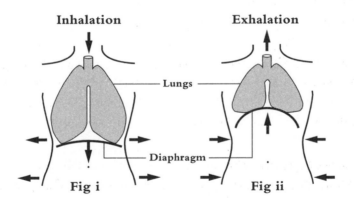

Learn to practise the Complete Diaphragm Breath lying down, sitting and standing. When it is familiar to you, practise it whilst you are walking (without your hand position) and just breathe more easily in rhythm with your steps. When you feel confident begin to change the rhythm of your breath slightly so that you breathe out for a little longer than you breathe in. Then develop it so that you hold the breath in, pausing momentarily, breathing out for a little longer, hold the breath momentarily – and continue in this way.

ii *The Complete Diaphragm Breath with arm movements*

This is to exercise the muscles in the chest, arms and back, to control the diaphragm, expand the capacity of the lungs and increase coordination and mental concentration.

i) Lie flat on your back with your arms by your sides with the backs of the hands flat on the floor beside your hips.

ii) Thoroughly exhale as you draw the abdomen in.

iii) Begin to practise your diaphragmatic breathing and as you breathe in move your arms out to the sides with the backs of hands and fingers touching the floor all the time – and reach above your head.

iv) Bring the arms and hands together and link the thumbs. As you hold the breath in for a moment notice the expansion deep into the *base* and *sides of the lungs*. Do this without straining.

v) Begin to draw the abdomen in as you slightly exhale bringing your arms back down by your sides in the same way with the fingers and backs of the hands touching the floor all the way down.

Repeat this three more times.
Make absolutely sure that the arm movements synchronise with the breath in order to gain maximum benefit.

iii *Chest opening*

The following exercise opens out the chest in a way that is particularly suitable for people who have a tendency to shallow breathing, tightness in the chest, bronchitis or asthma.

Please share this with anyone who has difficulty in breathing or tension in the chest. As a therapeutic posture it is invaluable. You can use cushions and pad for support so that you can stay in the position for longer as you breathe quietly, deeply and naturally.

a Unsupported – *see Fig (i)*

i) Lie flat on your back, legs straight, arms by your sides and chin tucked in.

ii) Take the weight on the elbows as you raise the head, neck and shoulders and lean back.

iii) Push up with the abdomen, solar plexus and chest in that order and, if it is right for you, tip the head back. Really open out the chest and throat deeply compressing the back of the neck. Bring the shoulders right back and avoid sinking in between them. Hold that position breathing naturally and notice how the air can reach the base and sides of the lungs.

iv) Raise the head, look at your feet and *ease* the spinal column into the floor from the back of the waist, in between the shoulder blades and then lower the head to the floor as in the original position.

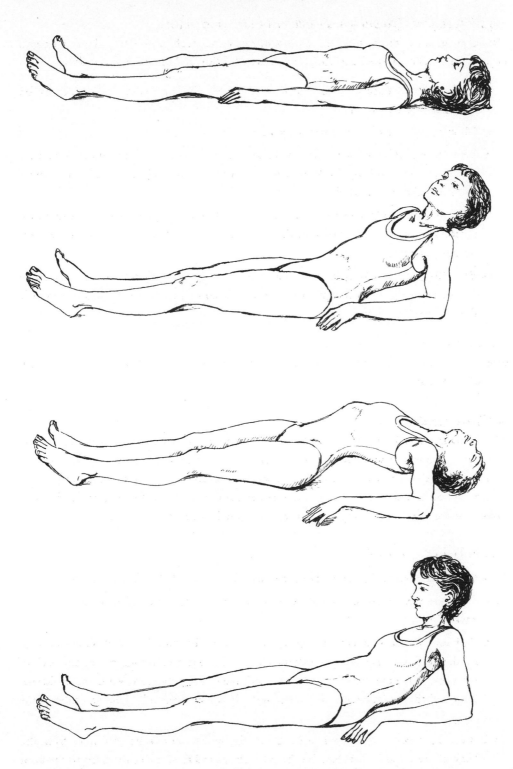

b **Supported** – *see Fig (ii)*

    i) Place the cushions or pads under the back just slightly above the waist. Make sure that you have enough support and height without straining.

    ii) Place another cushion to support the head slightly lower and the back if possible so that you can tip back, opening out the throat and relaxing the head, neck and shoulders.

    iii) Take the weight on the elbows and lean back over the cushions. Open the arms to the sides, so forming a cross, with the hands on the floor. Hold that position for a few minutes breathing deeply and evenly concentrating on the air reaching the depth and sides of the lungs.

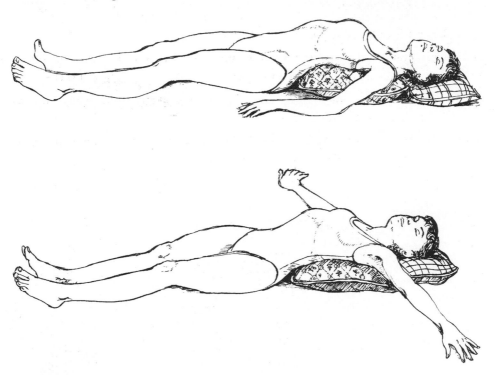

    iv) Open the mouth wide and take a deep breath into the chest as you swallow the air, close the mouth and breathe out of the nose. Repeat this twice more – and relax.

    v) Push the cushions out of the way and lie flat on the floor with arms by your sides and relax deeply enjoying the exhilarating effect in your chest.

Breathing in through the mouth and out of the nose in this dynamic way is particularly relevant to people who experience the fear of not being able to breathe during a panic attack. To bend back over a bed or sofa in this way at such a time can release that fear and return to norm more easily and gently.

    Tightness in the chest and difficulty in breathing can often be the result of suppressed emotions. After practising physical movement in this way, it is not unusual for emotional tension to be released in some way and this may be through feeling sad, overjoyed, upset or angry and needing to cry or laugh. Please accept that your body is working most beautifully for you and is doing its best for you on all levels. This highlights the powerful link between mind, body and emotions. If you wish to cry then go along with it. Fully accept the sadness and the thoughts and memories that are there, however long ago, and make the most of the opportunity to release them in a gentle non-threatening way. Accept it all in order to let it go.

iv *Square breathing*

This exercise increases breath retention and control, establishes a natural rhythm and increases mental concentration and powers of visualisation.

i) Take up the basic sitting position – and relax.

ii) Begin to notice the two main parts of the breath – inhalation and exhalation. Establish an even rhythm and allow the breath to stabilise.

iii) After you breathe out begin to count up to *four* for the inhalation – pause – and then to *four* for the exhalation – pause – and so on.

iv) Notice the two other parts of the breath – slight retention *after* the inhalation and *after* the exhalation, and begin to count to *two* for each.

v) Visualise a door frame – see Figure (i).

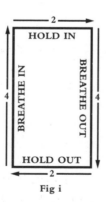

Fig i

Breathe in, count 4, from bottom left hand to top left hand corner.

Hold in, count 2, from top left hand corner to top right hand corner.

Breathe out, count 4, from top right hand to bottom right hand corner.

Hold out, count 2, from bottom right hand to bottom left hand corner.

Repeat this up to six times or until you have established an even flow.

vi) In order to progress and extend, change the shape from the rectangle of a door frame to the square of a tile on the wall (see Figure ii) and continue in the same way as you hold the breath in and out to the count of four, but do not strain to do that.

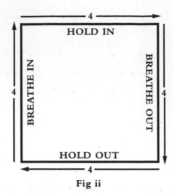

Fig ii

When you have established this well without straining you can extend the count from four to six. Practise this whilst you are walking too.

v Simple alternate nostril breathing

This wonderful, much celebrated technique is based upon the different effects that breathing through each nostril has upon all levels of our being. There is a whole science of balance within this structure – that of activity and passivity, masculinity and femininity and so on – the balance of opposing forces.

In natural healthy breathing there is a tendency for one nostril to have dominance over the other for a period of about one and a half to two hours. Wisdom of ancient medicine supports this in the belief that if the nostrils are out of kilter the whole person is vulnerable and susceptible to imbalance and disease – hence the tremendous interest in the alternate nostril breathing to regulate and balance. Scientific and medical experiment has recently shown that this balance between left and right nostrils has a direct bearing upon the acid/alkali and calcium/potassium balance within the body.

It is not good enough just to read these things and reject or accept them blindly. You can check this out for yourself in the following way:-

Throughout the day – say, on the hour and on the half hour, just check which nostril is more clear.

Sit quietly and let the breath stabilise.

i) close the right nostril with the thumb and just notice the air moving in and out of the body through the left nostril for several breaths. Notice how it feels then release the thumb.

ii) close the left nostril in the same way and notice the breath in as before – and let go.

You may notice that it is easier to breathe through one nostril than the other.

Do this every one and a half hours throughout the day and notice any changes in the ease or 'dis'ease of breathing through one or other or both and if it is highlighted by the warmth and coolness of your body and personality. Make a note of the pattern over a period of a week and a month.

The effects and benefits of the alternate nostril breathing are as follows. It clears and cleans the nasal passages and sinuses.

It balances the autonomic nervous system – the sympathetic active attitude and the parasympathetic passive attitude – and encourages the mind and emotions to become calm and evenly balanced. And it prepares the mind for further concentration.

i) Take up the basic sitting position.

ii) Thoroughly exhale out of both nostrils.

iii) ★Take up the hand position – right thumb over right nostril and breathe in through the left nostril slowly, evenly and deeply without straining. Just *allow* the breath to enter the lungs without trying too hard.

iv) When fully inhaled close the left nostril with the ring finger of the right hand, pause for a moment.

v) Release the thumb as you exhale out of the right nostril slowly, evenly and thoroughly.

vi) When fully exhaled and without straining, pause momentarily and without changing the hand position breathe in again through the right nostril evenly and deeply.

vii) When fully inhaled pause momentarily, closing the right thumb over the right nostril.

viii) Release the ring finger and breathe out of the left nostril thoroughly and evenly. Pause for a moment.

This represents one complete round. Repeat without straining from ★ for two more rounds.

Practise this on a daily basis – just three rounds each time until you feel quite ready to develop it to five rounds. After you have been practising five rounds for a few weeks gradually extend it to several minutes.

After each time just rest and be still for a while as this will have a natural calming effect. If you have the time then lie down and rest thoroughly for five or ten minutes.

It is most beneficial to practise this on a *regular daily basis* to have an accumulative effect rather than using it as a last resort to calm down. Let this technique gradually work its way into your system to balance your physical, mental and emotional make-up. This is far more beneficial than 'popping pills' in an attempt to reach the desired result for *it is you who is in charge* and not the pills.

vi *Recharging and directing the life-force*

The solar plexus is a centre of tremendous energy – a storehouse of life-force. In this exercise the aim is to tap into that source and direct it to other parts of the body to energise, recharge and ease tension and pain. In the process a feeling of tranquillity and calm may well come over you.

i) Lie down on the floor in the basic position and prepare for the complete diaphragmatic breath.

ii) Locate your navel and place your hands over your solar plexus so that the finger tips of each are just touching each other slightly above the navel. Have the palms of your hands flat against your body with elbows resting on the floor.

iii) Breathe easily, naturally and gently and contact this source of solar energy both physically and mentally. Begin to feel the build-up of energy in your finger tips and palms. Visualise it as a golden light.

iv) Choose where in your body you wish to direct this energy e.g. to anywhere that requires extra attention due to discomfort, tension or pain or to the head in order to generally recharge your batteries.

v) After the next inhalation transfer your hands to the area that you have chosen and exhale easily, naturally and gently, visualising that golden healing light entering the body at that place, flooding it with energy.

vi) After you have thoroughly exhaled replace your hands at your solar plexus and repeat this ten to fifteen times.

vii) When you have become familiar with the technique begin to include counting. For example, count ten for the inhalation with your hands at the solar plexus visualising light entering into your hands; count three whilst you hold the breath in and transfer your hands to the chosen area; count ten for the exhalation whilst you visualise the light flooding into that area; count three with the breath out whilst you return your hands back to the solar plexus – and so on.

Affirmations (see also page 39)

I am well blessed with healthy lungs.

Breathing deeply and calmly is coming easily to me now.

Deep even breathing now has a calming effect on all parts of my mind and body.

Life-force, radiant health and vitality are flowing to all parts of my body with every breath I take.

7 Food: Nourishment or Punishment

Eating, food and nutrition are relevant on all levels of your being. Food is anything that feeds you. The air that you breathe and the sun's life-giving rays are essential to you for without them you would not exist. You perceive and absorb through your senses which feed the mind, emotions and spirit.

Mental and emotional food

The mind, too, requires daily inspiration. Through your senses you can see beautiful and horrible creations – things that delight and offend the eyes; hear uplifting, exhilarating words and music or a cacophony of noises that grate; smell tantalising aromas or an offending stink; taste delicious flavours or something objectionable; touch velvet, satin, smooth skin, green moss or something that will make you creep. The mind is constantly being fed with a whole range of suggestions through conversation, other people, reading, the media, radio, television, press and the environment. The quality of these messages has a direct bearing upon your mental state.

Without love and comfort you can feel starved and neglected. The love that people share between each other is food. Some feel this is safer with household pets and other animals. Whatever the source, every human being has an emotional requirement to be fed with love and comfort. Eating food can act as compensation especially if it is something that you feel you should not have like chocolate, sweets, cream cakes and so on.

As well as survival there are many other reasons for eating. Parents nurture and comfort their children. In turn those same children may well play the same role with their ageing parents. We also eat through habit, to take a break, boredom, to stay awake, to change the mood, distract attention, etiquette, please other people, depression, tension – and so on. Food is used to please, nurture, treat, celebrate, reward, control and manipulate a situation or other people to our way of thinking.

During childhood food plays many roles which continue through adult life. When unwell you may have been given something special, lovingly prepared, and containing love and comfort to help you back to strength. In adult life you may be drawn towards them not only when you feel unwell but when you feel in need of love and comfort too. You may also be repelled by them – and not only because of the taste but the memory that is attached to it.

Do you remember the kind of feeling that you experienced when you did not wish to eat certain foods for which you had an instinctive dislike – was it cabbage, brussel sprouts, tripe and onions or semolina? Do you remember the reaction of the adults around you when you couldn't eat? What kind of feelings do you have now when you are faced with those foods?

Protection and insulation

Fat and *money* are very emotive words. They can both be the source of a great deal of comfort and stress. They represent a great store of energy and are used to insulate and protect. People crave them and despise them. Fat people are often regarded as jovial, happy and the best lovers. Whoever started these rumours were just maintaining the effective mask which can cover a deep dissatisfaction. Being fat or thin may comply with what we think is expected of us – it can also be an expression of rebellion against that expectation.

Our basic requirements are love, warmth, protection and security and the whole person sets out to establish these in one way or another. When one of these ingredients is absent or we fear that they may be so, we subconsciously aim to balance. Sometimes we go off our food and sometimes we overeat.

Fat

'No one will want me if I am fat'

This is a negative statement which comes from a poor self-image and lack of confidence. The psyche makes a statement which is played out by the body most brilliantly in order to support that feeling. It is substantiated by becoming fat which, in the eyes of the beholder, just proves the point of being unattractive and unlovable. Hence 'No one loves me'. The condition protects and insulates the person from other people. Even if the chance of a warm loving relationship or better job arises it may well be held with suspicion for the basic feeling of inadequacy is still there. Fat has met the supply and demand system that has been set up through negative programming of poor self-image, low self-esteem and lack of confidence.

'He only loves me when I am fat/thin/have blonde/black hair' etc.

In feeling unsure of oneself, it is reassuring to know that love and comfort are available from another person, albeit through gratifying that person's condition. Therefore the compliance is made – fat, thin, blonde or black hair etc – in order to secure the love and comfort at a cost.

Another form of protection and insulation takes place as a result of intrusion. It is not unusual for the psychic or fortune teller to put on weight as a subconscious form of protection against the bombardment of others' psychic energies.

Similarly, *starving* can be a way of punishing and bringing attention.

'If I don't eat, they will show that they care about me'
'If I get thin they will notice and worry about me'
'If I am sick they will have to look after me'

Fatness and thinness can therefore play a healthy and unhealthy part in maintaining a semblance of balance. Recognising the role being played by body size gives choice in the situation. In this respect any person who has genuine excess fat could ask themselves:

- Do I like my fat?
- Why is it there?
- Am I insulating or protecting myself from someone or something?
- Am I still living out that 'lovable, chubby puppyfat' child that had so much attention?
- Is this the only way I can get attention?
- Is it scarey to develop the real me?
- What am I hiding from myself and others?
- Am I using my fat to protect me from people getting too near me?
- What am I keeping back, hoarding in my gut and not letting go?

If any of this is relevant to you then give yourself time to answer these questions. Dwell upon them. If you choose to write what you are saying to yourself then do so creatively – almost without thought as though it is coming from the 'top of your head' rather than trying to work out a logical reply.

How you experience the world outside and beyond yourself is a true reflection of how you are within. If you feel vulnerable, unlikeable, unworthy and have a poor self-image you will be looking through those 'coloured spectacles' and everything you perceive and do will be coloured by them. Food and eating are used to compensate and balance at all levels. How much love and respect you have for yourself is reflected by how you treat your physical body. If you truly love and respect yourself and feel balanced throughout those levels the act of eating will be the act of nourishment and not punishment. You will begin to believe: I like and love myself unconditionally.

Spiritual food

Spiritual food is an essential part of man's nature. Many people through sheer enjoyment of life have the ability to touch something that is beautiful, invisible and intangible. For example, music can give rise to ecstasy and thanksgiving; great happiness can be experienced by being at one with Nature, the very pulse of life itself.

> *'To see a world in a Grain of Sand,*
> *And a Heaven in a Wild Flower,*
> *Hold Infinity in the palm of your hand,*
> *And Eternity in an hour'*

> (William Blake, *Auguries of Innocence*)

For some this is known as God, Divine Source, Deity, Light, Christ, Mohammed, Buddha, Universal Architect or Intelligence, Cosmic Motor – however and whatever It is conceived to be – label and no label.

LIVERPOOL
JOHN MOORES UNIVERSITY
AVRIL ROBARTS LRC
TEL. 0151 231 4022

'In any way that men love me in that same way they find my love for many are the paths of men but they all in the end come to me.

(Bhagavad-gita 4 : 11)

In *any* way – at work, play, with other people, alone, through reading, study, music, prayer, meditation, Nature, creativity and so on in countless ways – this awareness can come unbidden at any time – this divine presence which both feeds and requires feeding in order To Be.

Some people live to eat and may eat very well but it could be an interesting exercise for those people to imagine what a week would be like without eating – no planning, shopping, stocking, storing, preparation, cooking, eating and clearing away afterwards. It could be even more interesting to fast for a week in order to see what else there is in life.

If there is a depletion on the physical, mental, emotional or spiritual level of nourishment there is a subtle shift within all the levels in an attempt to balance that lack. When this happens it can manifest in overindulgence or starvation in any level in order to compensate. It is quick and easy to turn to physical food and overeating may be due to a lack of emotional comfort and love. The great need for physical touching may also be due to a lack of emotional touching. Spiritual poverty can lead to material greed, and vice versa, a bottomless pit which cannot be satiated. Nothing is separate – and so, in an attempt to balance the intake of food of every kind the need is often misplaced and there is a dive for the biscuit tin, cake tin or chocolate bar, a new household gadget, new relationship, new clothes, love almost at any cost, extra this or that, anything as long as it is quick, easy and immediately satisfies that pang. If you can accept this as a basis for eating it can bring a wider understanding and vision of *why* you eat and *what food is* to you.

Punishment

Eating patterns and food content affect, and are affected by, individual personality, attitude, awareness, family and social situation, culture and Mother Earth. Nature in her wisdom has provided us with all that we require and the more we get away from nature and natural rhythm the more we lose a sense of natural balance. Unnatural and inappropriate habits are developed and, even with an awareness of them, we still continue repeating them almost as though we are challenging or punishing ourselves. In the case of food it may be just to see how much we can stand – really punishing ourselves for example, too much junk food, alcohol, unbalanced diet – and then, bang! something happens to disturb the balance – overweight, underweight, allergy, illness, disturbed sleep pattern, overactive, nervous debility or change in character. 'What did I tell you' you say to yourself almost as though you needed to prove a point to yourself. This strange syndrome of denying and challenging the innate wisdom gets us into all kind of trouble. For most of us the opportunity for balance is in the imbalance for it is only when the weight problem or illness occurs that it is time to look at diet and nutrition.

Are you what you eat?

All matter has three qualities. In biophysics these are known as quarks and they exist in varying ratios according to the nature of the matter. These three qualities are referred to in *The Bhagavad-gita* and this is one way of viewing food that can help you make constructive choices about what to eat.

According to this ancient text, food has these three qualities in varying degrees and has a direct effect upon the person. Similarly, people have these three qualities and because of their personality will prefer foods of like nature.

Sattvic foods are of pure energy – such as fruit, vegetables, tomatoes, honey, dates, almonds and unrefined sugar, seeds, milk products and cereals – they are sweet, soft and nourishing. These foods are pure and light and help to clear and cleanse the system and give a feeling of lightness in body and mind. They promote life, vitality, health, joy and cheerfulness.

Rajsic foods are of high energy – hot, spicy, salty, red meat and alcohol and they can taste bitter, sour, pungent and harsh. They overheat the system which can lead to over activity – too much talking, being hot tempered, having strong likes and dislikes and love and hate passionately. A Rajsic diet can bring grief, pain and disease.

Tamsic foods are of low energy – overcooked, reheated, stodgy puddings, heavy meats, spoilt, tasteless, putrid, stale and unclean. Dry stodgy food can clog up the system and produce a feeling of heaviness and being dull, slothful and lazy.

These three qualities are never found in isolation. They are in a state of change and one can prevail over another at any one time.

Personal choice

In addition to being drawn towards particular kinds of foods you can also choose to eat the foods of either pure, high or low energy and therefore affect how you are. For example, people of high and low energy could eat more 'pure' foods in order to clear and cleanse the system and become lighter – not only in physical weight but in mental clarity.

You may like to check this out for yourself over a period of time. You could start by eating 'pure' foods for about ten days; then change to high energy foods for the next ten days; then change to low energy foods for the next ten days. Monitor your physical and mental tendencies. Through this experience you will begin to get to know how you like to feel and how you do not like to feel and what suits you.

Your choice of food has a direct bearing on your personality and whole wellbeing. In addition to that you can choose the foods that will suit your activities so that you will be at your best. You can then set about making definite choices not only of what you eat but how and what you want to be.

Food

A great deal of food is de-natured and highly refined with additives, colourants and preservatives. So much of it has been forced to grow beyond its natural rhythm and sprayed with insecticides, pesticides and glazing. It is tinned, frozen, hermetically sealed and presented in highly commercial packaging which refers to the manufacturer or packer rather than the beauty of the food itself. Even fruits arrive with a stamp of some organisation as though there is no credit awarded to the fruit itself – just the way in which it has been picked and presented.

Man seems to have developed a great lack of respect for food and its purpose. The polarities at work are the commercial world of massive profit and the great move towards more natural foods with a recognition of the effect that food can have on the physical body and mental state.

Food is big business and we are all highly affected by the opposite presentations of healthy eating and high consumer junk food. Music played in supermarkets is to seduce you into buying more than you need so avoid shopping when you are hungry for the same reason.

Diet and nutrition

There is a profusion of advice on diet and nutrition. What suits one person, however brilliantly, may not suit another. An imposed diet can be a hit and miss affair. It is up to you to seek out what is right for you, when it is right and for what reason rather than blindly following some fashionable craze. The human body is not just a mechanical engine with a boiler requiring stoking and firing.

The very word *diet* has developed a punitive quality inferring reducing, fat free, high fibre, gluten free, special foods for specific illness and so on. Diet is a way of eating – it is as simple as that. The reason for food is to build, sustain and repair the substance of the body and mind and to prevent and resist degenerative forces. Food is also a means of keeping body and soul together although the main emphasis seems to have little to do with the aspect of the soul.

A person concerned with diets may well say that the majority of allergy and illness is caused by faulty diet and constipation. Others may say – 'It is all in the mind' – purely psychological, psychosomatic. An environmentalist may say that it is as a result of pollution in the atmosphere. Others may say that all illness is a result of sickness of the spirit. All of these are right in their own way. Indeed diets can be crucial and essential part of healing. It is essential to aim at the development of true awareness and recognise what the body needs, does not need and just wants.

Life-force

Life-force exists in all living matter in varying degrees. The more life-force the higher quality of food. You can almost see the life-force in a bunch of fresh watercress or an orange as you peel it. You can almost sense the lack of it in something like tinned stuffed pork roll and pre-wrapped, processed and bleached foods. Eating high quality foods in moderate quantity in the right way can yield best nutritional results, whereas low quality foods in large proportions not eaten in the right way can lead to a form of deprivation and starvation.

Balanced diet

A good balanced diet consists of different components, including Protein, Carbohydrates, Fats, Fibre, Vitamins, Minerals and Water.

Fruit

All fruits have a natural sugar content, are a source of energy, fibre, include vitamins and minerals and have a cleansing effect. They are therefore an ideal food to form the basis of a diet rather than an extra, in between or just after meals. Sun-ripened fresh fruit is far more beneficial than tinned or frozen. Fruit is digested far more quickly than other food – but if it is eaten immediately after other food fermentation can take place in the stomach leading to a feeling of bloatedness.

Green vegetables

These include essential minerals and vitamins in more profuse quantity than other foods.

Raw food

Raw fruit and vegetables in their *natural* state include no additives. There is no depletion of vitamins and minerals through cooking, they provide first-class fibre, and are quick and easy to prepare.

Always wash fruit and vegetables well and aim to include them as a meal once a day.

Fresh food

Gather the freshest food available and be very discerning about pre-packed foods and date expiry. Frozen food can be excellent but watch the labels for content and additive. Tinned and packeted foods are third in life-force value.

Meat

More and more people are eating less and less meat for several reasons:

- most meat has added hormones and antibiotics with inevitable effects
- the ethical reason not to harm animals
- it is said that red meat coarsens the mind
- it produces a feeling of heaviness due to the amount of time that it takes to digest, let alone chew efficiently.

If you are a heavy meat eater why not try reducing or doing without it for a week or two and see how you feel? Then eat a steak or roast beef and notice the physical and mental effect. Experience is the best teacher.

Develop improved habits

If you decide that you wish to stop or reduce certain foods that have been part of your diet for a long time first become fully aware of your reason for doing so and recognise this as a conscious choice to enjoy and/or suffer without them. Do not suddenly cease eating them but rather fade them out of existence. Monitor how you feel and you will learn so much about what suits you in this way. Avoid altering your diet too drastically in too short a time and avoid extremes.

Rather than living by a list of dos and don'ts think about encouraging good food and discouraging inappropriate food.

Encourage and increase	Discourage and decrease
Raw sun-ripened fresh fruit	Tins and packets
	Additives
Raw fresh naturally grown salads and vegetables	Precooked
	Reheated
	Sauces and dressings
Fresh foods with maximum life-force	Overcooking
	Refined sugar and salt
Wholemeal bread	Puddings and pies
	Highly refined white bread
Plenty of water between meals	Strong tea and coffee
Fruit juice, delicious herb teas, hot water with a slice of lemon, mineral waters	Drinking when eating as this dilutes valuable digestive juices

When you are considering whether to treat (or punish yourself) to a chocolate bar, cream cake or cup of coffee etc. and you are having an argument with yourself as to the wisdom of it – try the tip of cleaning your teeth instead. You may find that this will alleviate the urge. However, if weighing up the pros and cons you decide to go ahead and 'munch' or 'slurp' *enjoy it totally rather than feeling guilty* – it is a far healthier attitude.

Train yourself to become aware of the life-force and nutritional value of foods *before you eat them*.

Keep it simple. You could spend all day preparing an exotic dish that looks fantastic but has very little nutritional value and is difficult to digest.

Avoid eating too late. The time between mid-evening and morning is for rest and repair. Energy is required for eating and if you eat too late these two processes become at loggerheads with each other, resulting in poor digestion and poor sleep.

Eat outside in the fresh air as much as you can as the flavour of food is enhanced.

Appetite. Trust your *natural desire* of hunger and thirst. It is very easy to eat for other reasons. The more you eat the more you will want to eat and conversely, the less you eat the less you will want to eat.

Overcooking reduces and destroys life-force, minerals, vitamins and flavour. An attempt is then made to recapture the flavour by adding more salt or sugar etc.

Be aware of eating twice

- 'I haven't eaten all day so I'll just grab a cheese sandwich or piece of cake whilst preparing dinner'
- Eating tea with the children and dinner with your partner
- Cosy snacks around the TV or fire during the middle of the evening can become a social habit in spite of having eaten a good dinner
- 'I can't bear waste' as you hover around the fridge, second helpings and leftovers
- 'Eating for two'

Speed. In a busy life quick, easy meals have an appeal. Speed does not necessarily mean lack of quality and nutrition, for what could be quicker than eating raw fruit and vegetables in their natural state of goodness.

Only partially fill the stomach rather than eating until you are no longer hungry as the digestive process takes time.

Visualise. Just now and again before eating look at your food and visualise its journey through your body and the effect that it will have. If you have chosen good highly nutritious food you will immediately feel good but if you have chosen food of poor quality you will realise the adverse effect that it could have.

High quality. As you eat high quality food visualise the life-force flowing throughout your body.

Additives

There is a vast variety of additives used in mass produced foods. They preserve, colour, flavour, bind together, separate, moisten and dry out. Denatured, highly processed, refined foods are artificially flavoured to compensate for the lack of flavour as a result of the process.

The known harmful effects include allergies, skin irritation, cold symptoms, catarrh, bowel disturbance, obesity, blurred vision, headaches, palpitations, nervous debility, lethargy, depression, hyperactivity, change in blood pressure and so on. Some can cause the thyroid glands to enlarge due to iodine content and handling of the dyes has been linked with skins cancer. Some of these additives are found in seemingly innocent foods like fish fingers, smoked fish, biscuits, scotch eggs, ice cream, bottled sauces, custard powder, gravy granules, crisps, cheese spread and margarine. The greatest damage to physical and mental health is not necessarily air pollution, violence or nuclear threat but the very food that we put in our mouths in the form of supposed nourishment. We could spend all our time trying to dodge additives and chemicals and end up in confusion, not caring, feeling guilty, or going off eating altogether.

It is essential to find out as much as you can about additives from a reliable source and then watch the labels. It is up to everyone to take responsibility for themselves and not only rely upon the troubleshooters.

Allergy

Why is it that, after years and years, someone suddenly develops an allergy to something in their diet? What a relief it is to find the source of that allergy, avoid it and regain a sense of balance. But how long before that imbalance re-appears as a result of something else. Maybe this allergy is a cry from the very core of our being which is yelling out – 'Enough is enough! Look at *me*, listen to me, touch me, feel me, look at what is happening. I feel so scared and frightened and there is nothing I can do but retreat. Can't touch this, can't touch that. Can't eat this, can't eat that.' In an attempt to survive we become more and more precious but in so doing that precious quality can be our very downfall. It is difficult and virtually impossible to avoid absorbing some of the additives that creep into our food, polluted atmosphere and the negative conditioning through the media. In order to survive and become more immune it is necessary to absorb a certain amount in order to survive and become a part of the world in which we live.

Fasting

'Everyone has a doctor in him' wrote Hippocrates. 'We just have to help him in his work . . . to eat when you are sick is to feed your sickness.'

Animals have the wisdom to stop eating when they are unwell in order to conserve their energy and mobilise their own healing powers. In every religion fasting has been a ritual. Fasting is particularly relevant to stress and tension and can successfully be used to:

- rest and cleanse the system to feel lighter and clearer physically, mentally and emotionally
- lose weight
- overcome craving and desire for food
- reduce drug dependency, alcohol and cigarette smoking
- lower high blood pressure and cholesterol level
- assist the *natural* healing process
- reduce tension and improve sleep
- as preparation prior to starting a project
- increase self discipline
- experience a heightened sense of spiritual awareness.

Bonuses are looking and feeling better and saving time and money.

No food is taken in a fast – only water. Fasting is *not* starving. When you stop eating the body continues to release toxins and waste material. The tongue becomes coated, the breath has an acetone odour and you may have a headache or feel dizzy due to lowered blood pressure. If you have a tendency to aches and pains they may be highlighted at the beginning of the fast. These are all healthy signs that the flushing is taking place. This is definitely the time *not* to stop as the fast is really beginning to work – just keep drinking plenty of water to encourage the flushing.

Between the last food at night and the first food in the morning there is a natural time of fasting – hence the word *breakfast*. This period can be extended to one or two days a week, several days a month or several weeks according to the reason and aim of the fast. Attitude is crucial. Think of the fast as a celebration of the body rather than punishing it. Focus on the positive signs of looking and feeling better.

General hints on fasting

- Start with just one or two days a week and when you feel ready extend that to three to five days once a month. When the tongue is clear, the breath clean, the eyes bright and you feel really good, decide whether you wish to finish the fast or continue and for how long. Remind yourself of your original reason and assess the benefits so far.

- Drink at least eight pints of mineral water a day preferably at room temperature rather than ice cold from the fridge. Keep to water only – no coffee, tea, juice or alcohol. Please do not smoke.

- Allocate your eight pints first thing in the morning. Consider anything over that a bonus.

- Buy a good mineral water. Tap water has additives that your refined taste buds will detect. Do not use mouthwash or toothpaste as they too have additives.

- Drink out of your best cut glass or fine bone china tea cup if it gives you extra pleasure.

- Every day exercise well, have plenty of fresh air and sunshine if possible. Take a shower or bath – the skin is the largest organ of secretion and needs flushing from the outside too.

- You may well interpret the gnawing feelings from your stomach as hunger but this is the body adjusting to a reduced workload. Sip water to reduce the feeling of hunger.

- If you are on regular medication please ask your doctor's advice.

- Fast to celebrate rather than punish.

- Avoid sudden movement as lowered blood pressure may make you feel dizzy.

- Fasting with others can give you encouragement and support.

- If in doubt please consult your doctor.

Caution

Please do not fast without your doctor's blessing if you are very thin, elderly, pregnant or have any kind of chronic condition or physical disease.

Are you how you eat?

Health comes from within and although the body is constructed from the foods eaten we are also a result of *how* the body and mind assimilate.

The quality of preparation and presentation of food is also absorbed. 'I can't swallow that' and 'That makes me feel sick' are expressions used for food and feelings. Consider going hungry rather than eating food that has been prepared and presented with anger.

Hurry and worry are key ingredients for poor digestion. If you cook with your head in a stew you may end up with indigestion.

Food that has been prepared and presented with love and care is food well blessed and Kirlian photography shows an increased life-force pattern in such food.

Mealtimes are used to catch up with the news through the TV, radio or press; watch a good programme on TV; read a good book; business planning and organisation; socialise; air grievances etc. Sometimes it is as well for the serrated edged knife to be in the guest's back rather than the steak for the amount of true goodness that is being done. No wonder it is difficult to 'swallow' the food sometimes, let alone what someone is saying across the table.

The external environment which you create for the consumption of food has a direct effect upon your internal environment. If there are ongoing disagreements that are highlighted at mealtimes think about calling a truce. You may find that this will improve your digestion and could shift rigid attitudes. Be honest with yourself and ask what you use food and mealtimes for. Make changes if necessary, for you are absorbing not only the food but the whole atmosphere.

Chewing

Digestion begins before food enters the mouth. Smell and thought encourage the digestive juices to flow. The quality of digestion relies a lot upon what happens in the first few inches of the digestive tract – mouth, teeth and tongue.

Always sit in a good upright position if possible as slumping in a chair does not help digestion. Energy is required to eat and the circulation of blood is drawn away from the extremities and towards the gut. It is therefore not unusual for someone frail, elderly or unwell to feel quite cold immediately after eating.

Flavours are released in the mouth and the taste buds begin to draw on the nutritional value. The tongue absorbs life-force. According to Ayurvedic medicine food has six flavours and all of them should be present in proportion in order to keep the body healthy and free from disease. The sweet, astringent and bitter foods are of a cool potency; sour, pungent and salty foods are of the hot potency. Each flavour has a specific task which involves stimulating certain organs to work efficiently.

The jaw, teeth, tongue and the action of chewing are an essential part of good digestion and nutrition – an opportunity to gain the maximum benefit from whatever quality food. Lack of nutrition and a feeling of starvation can be the result of ignoring this fact even with good quality food.

Ideally food should be chewed until it almost swallows itself. In this way you will not require the same quantity. Why not try for yourself – masticate your food until you gain maximum flavour. Wait until it is almost swallowed by itself. It is a whole new experience to check out. Experiment with something quite bland like a piece of dry bread and savour the flavour. Eating in this way can become fascinating as your taste buds will naturally require less additional flavour of salt, pepper and sugar. A single nut eaten in this way can be more nourishing than a whole bag which is bolted. Do remember that raw food takes longer to chew properly. Anyone with dental problems and dentures must take particular care to adjust the diet accordingly and chew well before swallowing in order to avoid indigestion and poor nutrition.

Guidelines

Respect yourself

Prepare and serve with care

Eat in a happy relaxed atmosphere

Chew thoroughly

Only partially fill the stomach

Rest after meals if only for five minutes

Have regular but not rigid meal times

Rely on your *natural* appetite

Moderation in all things – components and quantity

Learn as much as you can, put it into action and avoid becoming a fanatical bore

Let your body's intuition and innate wisdom guide you.

8 Body Posture and Exercise

Posture

'Stand up straight'

'Put your feet together'

'Hands out of your pockets'

'Chin up'

'Big boys don't cry'

'You're a big girl now – no need for that'

How often have you heard any or all of this and how often have you complied in some measure? These are attempts to convince others and often ourselves that something is not as it is – a gesture to hide feelings and a posture to convey a sense of being in control.

Mind and body are two parts of one whole enjoying, and suffering, a relationship of the most intimate kind. Feelings of joy, ecstasy, amusement, pain, sorrow, grief, anger and frustration are reflected in the body. It is impossible to be absolutely consumed with joy or anger without that being reflected physically. Posture has a direct bearing upon mental health and the stress of living can cause stiff, tight, rigid muscles.

The body speaks volumes without uttering a word. Your posture and the way you move has a direct effect upon how you are and what you feel. Changing physical posture can change mental and emotional posture.

If someone arrives for an interview with a 'hang-dog' expression, chest sunk in, feet and knees turned in, they might just as well complete the picture and verbally apologise for being there or, worst still, apologise for being at all.

The same person could arrive with an upright, open and relaxed chest, shoulders relaxed with head up and have a vastly different effect as they almost say with the open countenance 'This is me and I am pleased to be here now and prepared for what is to come'.

'Stand up straight' is intended to create an uprightness of thought where feelings do not get in the way and to give the impression of being totally in control. However, if this is not really so, you cannot fool yourself for very long and your body will soon begin to tell you through a build-up of tension. This may be felt through headaches, neck and shoulder pain, twitching, back pain, indigestion, palpitations and so on. If you *genuinely* feel good you genuinely look good and vice versa. This has little to do with physical attributes and beauty; it is a glowing from within – an inner beauty which has a therapeutic effect for self and others.

Physical and mental tension literally 'sits' in the body in different places for different people according to personality. Familiar key areas for discomfort and pain caused by tension are shoulders, neck, face, eyes, jaw, back, hands, stomach and chest. There are specific exercises later in this chapter which are devoted in particular to these areas that harbour tension.

Polite civilised Western woman has been taught to keep her legs crossed, wear tight skirts, have a nipped in waist and wear high-heeled shoes. Habitually crossing the legs is detrimental to the circulation and the whole posture. It also cuts off access to power and locks it in. Wearing tight skirts with nipped in waist encourages shallow breathing in the mid and upper chest only and disempowers the person from a sense of the earth. Most of the weight is naturally on the middle to back of the feet. High-heeled shoes plummet the body forward on to the front of the feet and unbalance the spinal column.

Poor posture can develop over a period of years and can lead to moving in an awkward and ungraceful manner. It can lead to discomfort and imbalance and is at the root of a lot of cases of poor breathing and indigestion.

Adjusting the posture

i) Raise the shoulders up as high as possible. Hold that position for a while very tense – then drop the shoulders down as far as possible, then back as far as possible with the shoulder blades toward each other, then forward as far as possible rounding the back and allowing the chest to sink in. Create as much movement in the shoulders as you can.

Roll the shoulders up, back, down and forward several times.

Change – roll the shoulders the other way several times – forward, down, back and up several times.

Then just let the shoulders settle and feel the warm exhilarating effect of those movements. Lengthen the back of the neck by tucking the chin in slightly and allow the head to settle.

ii) Using a mirror stand sideways and place your right hand on your abdomen. Place the left hand (palm out) on the small of your back. Manipulate the body by drawing the stomach in, while flattening the small of the back at the same time. Keep this position in a relaxed way whilst sitting, standing and walking.

iii) Stand with your back against the wall with heels, buttocks, shoulder blades and back of the head touching the wall. Avoid being too rigid. Step away from the wall retaining that line. As you walk let the feet and legs carry the body weight in a symmetrical way – feet pointing forward and not in or out.

iv) The carriage of the body is improved by stretching and this also reduces the tendency to shrink with the onset of years.

Holding onto a high rail or branch of a tree with your hands, feet off the ground and hanging will do wonders for your back, easing and stretching the tension away. Using a door jamb or bannisters will suffice but do not put yourself at risk.

Exercise

Mental and nervous tension, worry and anxiety deplete the physical substance and tense muscles trap valuable life-force. Exercise practised regularly can help to unlock tension by de-programming negative habits of stiffness and rigidity and keep it at bay. Research shows that physical exercise reduces the risk of stress. Physical and mental attitudes begin to shift and change to develop more strength, suppleness, stamina and resilience.

Lack of exercise and tiredness

Lack of exercise becomes obvious when you are surprised by becoming out of breath as a result of exerting yourself in a way which previously did not cause that to happen – climbing stairs or walking up a hill. You may well develop stiffness and discomfort generally or become overweight, feel tired and 'not at one' with yourself – as though you are sitting uneasily in your body.

Being naturally tired can be a result of lack of sleep or over exertion and the most natural way to cope with that is to rest and have more sleep. To ignore it or take pep pills and other stimulants in order to cope challenges your resources and natural rhythm. Not taking enough care of yourself at this stage can lead to chronic fatigue, exhaustion and lower your resistance. Although the body is capable of tremendous feats and can do without sleep for several days it is necessary to balance that exertion with deep rest. Please refer to the chapter on relaxation for the most efficient and satisfying form of restful awareness and deep rest.

If chronic fatigue is present it is wise to seek medical advice as it can be a symptom of an underlying cause.

Suitable exercise

A good maxim is to aim to get out of breath at least once a day, even if it is only running up and down stairs several times or running for the bus. Whenever possible walk rather than using car or bus.

The body is capable of being supple, strong and resilient. Each of these three components are developed in varying degrees with different activities -

Suppleness – allows you to be at ease with your body, flexible enough to stretch and bend, rather than rigid and prone to knocks, bumps and accidents.

Strength – muscle power is required to bear and resist weight and to push and pull.

Stamina – is required to withstand pressure over a period of time. Strong heart muscles provide stamina and resilience.

There are mountainous areas in the Andes of South America, Himalayas of India and Caucasus in Russia where many people live well over one hundred years. From early childhood these people walk steep paths inhaling pure mountain air, purifying cells and increasing life-force – strengthening legs, heart and lungs developing their stamina and the whole constitution.

A competitive spirit can be very fine and it can also be lethal when it creates psychological

LIVERPOOL
JOHN MOORES UNIVERSITY
AVRIL ROBARTS LRC
TEL. 0151 231 4022

tension of 'I'll beat them if it kills me' attitude – for it may well do. The only comparison of any real value in the aim to *improve and develop yourself is how you were, how you are* and *how you hope to be*. This attitude reduces false vanity. Exercises of this nature should not be confused with highly competitive sport. Sport needs time and may not fit in with an already busy life. An ideal form of exercise is one that makes you feel as though your body is 'singing'.

The following non-competitive exercises provide plenty of scope:

walking	cycling	Yoga
jogging	swimming	keep fit
running	dancing	martial arts
hill walking	disco dancing	

The rewards of good and appropriate exercise can be *seen physically* and *felt psychologically*. There is an improvement of:

- complexion and general appearance
- natural sleep and appetite
- resilience therefore strengthening the immune system
- release of tension and developing calmness
- self-confidence, self-awareness, self-image.

THE EXERCISE PROGRAMMES

The following programmes are aimed to stretch and ease tension out of the body and to build strength and stamina. Each programme is balanced so that the positions and movements complement each other. It is therefore recommended to keep to the suggested order.

Practised on a regular basis you can expect to experience:

- improved cardiovascular action of circulation and breathing
- increased suppleness
- release of tension
- increased energy
- improved concentration, co-ordination and balance.

i WAKE UP YOUR MIND AND BODY *Five to fifteen minutes*
Start the day as you mean to carry on with this celebrated and most famous Yoga routine – *Salutation to the Sun*.

ii **OFFICE ROUTINE** *Twenty minutes*

Take a break in the office to ease and stretch out tension and feel more energised and relaxed. This is also suitable for people with restricted or limited body movement whether of a temporary or more permanent nature.

iii **SPECIAL NEEDS** *Fifteen minutes*

A set of suggestions to ease tension out of specific areas – can be practised separately at any time during the day and with any of the above programmes.

General suggestions

- Wear loose unrestricting clothing and remove your shoes

- Choose an environment conducive to exercise

- Practise at a time when you are not likely to be interrupted – at least two hours after a light meal. Good times are

    - first thing in the morning to set you up for the day.

    - returning home from work to ease tension out of the day

    - at bedtime to ensure a good night's sleep

- Practise on a regular basis at a regular time. There is no progress without practice. Reading about exercise is not the exercise itself. Establish a positive habit daily if possible or at least three times a week. The more you practise the more you will experience benefit. Discipline is your friend here – remind yourself why you want to exercise and simply say to yourself 'Do it'. Treat it as taking a daily walk. Using exercise cassettes increases the discipline that is required for regular practice.

- Rest and relax after every exercise session so that you gain maximum benefit from your efforts. Please refer to the Complete deep relaxation on page 121.

Breathing

First become familiar with the physical movement and then include the specific breathing suggestions which are in *italics*. If in doubt, *leave it out* and just let the body take over naturally.

It is important to *move to the breath rather than breathe to the movement*. Holding of the breath in or out for an extended period of time is not advisable in cases of high blood pressure or if you experience unpleasant pressure in any way. Please take what is relevant for you and leave the rest.

If in doubt please check with your doctor.

i WAKE UP YOUR MIND AND BODY

Start the day as you mean to carry on with this celebrated and most famous Yoga routine – Salutation to the Sun. This is a series of twelve different postures traditionally practised facing the early morning sun as it rises in the east. It is a complete technique in itself and there are many variations. Its virtues are extolled at length by many. Many conditions are relieved including backache, constipation, digestive ailments, lumbago, muscular rheumatism, hypertension and fatigue. This is an excellent limbering up exercise that requires and improves mental alertness, balance and concentration.

Effects

- Tones digestive and elimination systems through massage of the viscera of liver, stomach, spleen, intestines and kidneys.
- Tones the nervous system by alternately stretching, bending and relaxing the spine which houses the central nervous system.
- Tones the endocrine gland system – regulating hormone release in the blood stream.
- Increases the efficiency of the cardio-vascular system. The lung capacity is increased and respiration is improved. Circulation is improved generally.
- Tones the muscles throughout – strengthening and rendering suppleness in joints.
- Back, legs and arms are stretched and strengthened.
- Removes psychosomatic tensions and blocks.

Start to compose the mind and body by being still

Sit in simple cross-legged posture on the floor. Close your eyes and relax from the top of the head down through the whole length of the body to the extremities of the fingers and toes. Just be still for a while. When ready, stand up and prepare to practise *Salutation to the Sun*. (See next page for illustration)

i) Stand tall, feet together, palms of the hands together in front of the chest.

ii) Raise the arms up and bend back from the waist.

iii) Stretch up tall and bend forward from the hips. Place the palms of your hands flat on the floor beside the feet, bending the knees if you need (the hands remain in this position throughout the sequence).

iv) Stretch the right leg back behind you as far as you can and tuck the toes under onto the floor. Lower the right knee to the floor and look up. Have the left thigh in contact with your abdomen/chest so creating a deep compression.

v) Bring the left foot back to join the right keeping the back parallel to the floor - known as the plank position.

vi) Lower the knees, chest and forehead onto the floor. Have the chest between the hands, bottom up, deeply curving the back of the waist without the abdomen touching the floor.

vii) Lower down completely – and relax.

viii) Raise the head, neck and shoulders, deeply curving the lower back and opening out the chest. Keep hips and lower abdomen on the floor, elbows bent and shoulders relaxed not hunched.

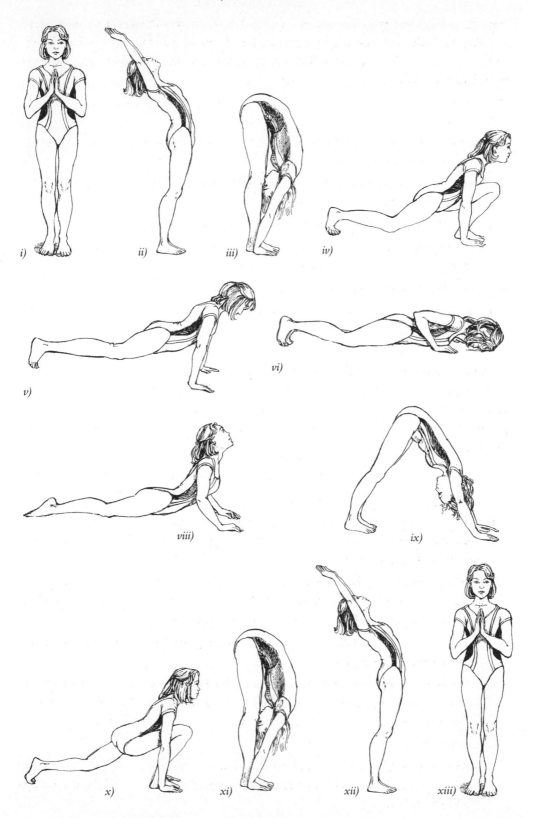

i)

ii)

iii)

iv)

v)

vi)

viii)

ix)

x)

xi)

xii)

xiii)

ix) Curl toes under and push up into a triangle shape, bottom up, heels towards the floor and head down between the arms, looking at your feet.

x) Look at the space between the hands and aim to bring the right foot flat on the floor to that space so that the right thigh creates a compression deep into chest and abdomen. If the foot does not reach that space bring it up as high as you can towards it. Left knee on floor if possible.

xi) Bring the left foot up to join the right. Straighten both legs really stretching the lower back and hamstrings.

xii) Raise your head and raise your arms out first and come up. Open out and stretch your arms back, deeply curving the back.

xiii) Resume the original position standing tall with feet together and palms of the hands together.

Practise the above until you are familiar enough with it to include the correct breathing as follows:

i Stand tall – *breathe out*

ii Raise the arms up – *breathe in*

iii Bend forward – *breathe out*

iv Stretch the right foot back – *breathe in*

v Bring the left foot to join the right – *hold the breath in*

vi Lower the knees, chest and forehead to the floor – *hold the breath in*

vii Lower on to the floor completely – *breathe out*

viii Raise the head, neck and shoulders – *breathe in*

ix Push up into triangle shape – *hold the breath in*

x Bring the right foot up – *hold the breath in*

xi Bring the left foot up to join the right – *breathe out*

xii Raise the head, stretch arms in front and come up – *breathe in*

xiii Resume the original position as you *breathe out*

When you have completed the practice of *Salutation to the Sun* lie down on your back in the *Basic Lying Position*, (see Appendix) and deeply relax. Close your eyes and become aware of your heart pumping energy around the body positively affecting all parts. Feel the body pulsating in rhythm to the vibration of your heart and enjoy the feeling of elation and revitalisation.

Take care in getting up from the floor.

Development

- When you are familiar with the physical positions begin to develop the suggested breathing pattern to enhance the whole procedure and increase its efficiency.

- Then practise three rounds.

- In time you can gradually increase to six rounds. At this stage in order to maintain balance please alternate each round with the leg movements so that, for example:

  Round one – *right leg stretches back in step 4) and forward in step 10)*

  Round two – *left leg stretches back in step 4) and forward in step 10)*

  Round three – right leg

  Round four – left leg . . . and so on.

- Gradually increase to twelve rounds.

Practised in an energetic way one round may take twenty seconds. At this rate you could be practising twelve rounds in four minutes! Do not be put off – take it all in your own time carefully developing what is right for you.

- Alternatively practise this routine for five minutes every day followed by five minutes relaxation. Gradually extend to ten minutes and then fifteen minutes. Practising in this way *you will know precisely how long you are going to devote to exercise.*

Practise this wonderful exercise in accordance with how you feel.

Some days you might feel like being very energetic as though you are pumping energy around the body. Another day you may prefer to practise smoothly, gracefully and calmly – take what is appropriate for you and when.

ii OFFICE ROUTINE

Take a break to ease, stretch and feel more energised and relaxed. The movements are described from sitting in an upright chair with feet flat on the floor, supported if necessary. They can equally be done standing. The programme is included in the tape entitled *Relax and Move Gently* from *Mind Your Body Cassettes.* (see Further Listening)

These techniques have also been chosen for their therapeutic value and have been found beneficial by many people, aged eight to eighty and with varying degrees of mobility and immobility. People who have arthritis, back pain, high blood pressure, arteriosclerosis, multiple sclerosis, polio and other disabling conditions have used these techniques and found them most helpful.

Regular practice can help to improve and maintain

- suppleness of joints
- elasticity of muscles
- efficiency of circulation and respiration.

As a very general rule it is good to keep the body moving. Narrow margins exist between stretch and strain, genuine tiredness and apathy and only you know how far you can go. It

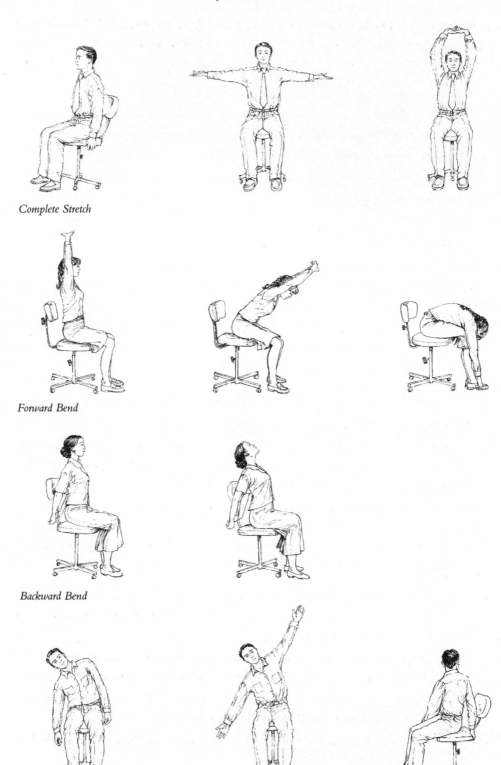

Complete Stretch

Forward Bend

Backward Bend

Sidways Bend

Twist

is totally up to the individual to ascertain what is right for themselves. If inflammation or real pain are present then rest is preferable. If in doubt please consult your doctor. There is no prize for contortion which causes pain. Please take each movement as far as is appropriate enjoying the energising and relaxing effect.

1 Complete stretch × 3

2 Forward bend × 3

3 Complete stretch and forward bend combined × 3

4 Backward bend × 3

5 Sideways stretch × 2

6 Twist × 2

7 Forward bend

8 Head, neck and shoulders

9 Feet, ankles and legs

10 Complete stretch

11 Rest

1 *Complete stretch*

i) Sit tall arms down by the side of the chair; legs slightly away from each other.

ii) Raise the arms out to your sides palms uppermost and stretch.

iii) Raise the arms up and over your head *breathe in*, link the thumbs together if you can. If this is not possible at the moment just keep your arms parallel to the floor. Take what is right for you. Hold the position *breathing naturally*.

iv) Lower the arms down by the side of the chair and *breathe out*.

Repeat twice.

2 *Forward bend*

i) Sit tall arms down by your sides. Have your feet slightly in front in order to support you but if the feet do not reach the floor have them supported with cushions or books. Raise the chin up and *breathe in*.

ii) Lean forward from the hips without collapsing in the chest. Aim to keep a long straight line from the top of your head to the base of the spine. *Breathe out*.

iii) Just let your arms hang in front of you. Rest your abdomen on your thighs. Relax the head down and just *hang* there. Rest and *breathe naturally*.

iv) When ready, raise the head and come back up placing the hands on the knees or sides of the chair if you need to. *Breathe in*.

v) Sit tall, *breathe out* – and let go.

Repeat twice more.

3 *Complete stretch and forward bend combined*

i) Sit tall and thoroughly *exhale*.

ii) Raise the arms up and out to your sides as you *breathe in*. Continue to stretch up and over the head if it is appropriate for you and link the thumbs and lift – really stretching tall.

iii) Hold that stretch for a while *breathing naturally*.

iv) Keeping the hands together, lean forwards from the hips as before. Aim to keep a long straight line from the base of the spine to the tips of the fingers.

v) Stretch forward and down with the trunk eased over the legs, *exhale*. Just *hang* and completely let go, feeling that wonderful s-t-r-e-t-c-h along the whole length of the back. Let the arms go, let your head be quite loose and *breathe naturally*.

vi) Raise the head and come up in the same way. Stretch the arms out in front of you, thumbs linked together. If you need help to come up place the hands either on the knees or on the sides of the chair. Breathe in. Sit tall – and let go.

Repeat twice more.

4 *Backward bend*

i) Sit tall and bring your arms around the back of the chair. Clasping your hands together if possible.

ii) Begin to open out the chest as you lean back, well supported by the chair, and tip the head back if it is right for you. Hold the position *breathing naturally*.

iii) Release the hands, raise the head back to centre and sit tall bringing the hands to rest on your lap. Drop the head down, tuck the chin in and just rest for a moment.

Repeat twice more.

5 *Sideways stretch*

i) Sit tall with feet firmly supported.

Slide the left hand and arm down the left side of the chair without leaning forward.

ii) Raise the right arm up and turn the head to look at the right hand. Hold that position *breathing naturally*. Lift the right arm up just a little further, *breathe in*, and as you lower it come back up to sitting tall and *breathe out*. Repeat to the right side.

Repeat the whole process once more each side.

6 *Twist*

i) Sit tall, feet firmly supported .

ii) Twist to the left. Bring the left arm behind the chair and grasp it with the hand if you can, using it as a lever to pull you round without straining. Turn the head to look over the left shoulder. Bring the right arm in front of you and take hold of the left side of the chair if you can – no straining. Hold that position *breathing naturally* and easily for several breaths.

iii) Bring the head back to centre and arms back by your sides – let go. Repeat with the right side.

Repeat the whole process once more each side.

7 *Forward bend*

Ease the back now by repeating the forward bend as already described. Just relax forward and allow the head and arms to hang, gently stretching the whole length of the spinal column.

When ready to come up, raise the head and place the hands on your knees or sides of chair for support if you need.

Breathe in, sit tall, and let go.

8 *Head, neck and shoulder exercises*

Now is a good time to practise these exercises as described in the Special Needs Section.

9 *Feet, ankles and leg muscles*

If you have not already done so please remove your shoes, socks or stockings and *let your feet breath!*

i) Sit tall having the thighs well supported by the chair.

ii) Raise the left foot up as you breathe in and push the heel away as much as you can, open out your toes. Tighten up the calf, knee and thigh muscles. Hold that position without straining. Check that you are not tightening up your arms, shoulders or jaw. Lower the leg breathing out – and rest.

Repeat that twice more with the left leg.

Repeat the whole process with the right leg three times.

iii) Raise the left foot up. Rotate the foot and ankle clockwise four times and then anti-clockwise four times – and lower.

Repeat with the right foot three times.

10 Bring the session to a close with the Complete Stretch twice more.

11 Just rest and relax for a while either sitting on the chair or lying flat on the floor.

iv SPECIAL NEEDS

Ease tension out of specific areas of your body.

These exercises can be practised separately at any time during the day and with any of the previous programmes.

1 Neck
2 Shoulders
3 Eyes
4 Jaw
5 Fingers, hands and wrists
6 Hand massage.

1 *Neck*

Sit or kneel in the *Basic Sitting Position* (see page 142). Sit tall and become aware of the back of the neck as part of the spinal column which starts where you are sitting and ends just below the base of the skull. In order to get the best from these exercises it is preferable to remain sitting upright. Start by slumping over and notice how the whole shape of the spine changes – rounded upper back, protruding chin, compression just below the base of the skull – then sit tall and relaxed with the shoulders down and chest open.

i) Close the eyes. Turn the head to the right as far as possible and then to the left. Do this several times and allow the movement to become quicker and quicker until you can really release the head and neck. Check that the jaw is relaxed. Have a picture in your mind of a dog after a swim just shaking his head from side to side. Bring the head back to centre.

ii) Looking straight ahead drop the head to the left – left ear towards the left shoulder without tensing the shoulder in any way – and then to the right. Do this up to twice more.

iii) Drop the head down tucking the chin well in and notice how far down into the upper back you experience that stretch. Tilt the head right up and back, keeping the shoulders relaxed. Open the mouth as wide as you can and relax the jaw. Then keeping the head in that position close the mouth and raise the head back up to centre. Repeat the forward and backward bend twice.

iv) Drop the head down, relax the jaw and rotate the head to the right so that the right ear faces the right shoulder – then drop forward again and to the left with the left ear toward the left shoulder. Repeat twice.

2 *Shoulders*

i) Hunch the shoulders right up underneath the ears. *Breathe in, hold that position and the breath* for a moment. Then quite forcibly drop the shoulders down *sighing deeply* out of the mouth as though you are releasing a heavy burden from your shoulder. Repeat twice.

ii) Rotate both shoulders in a clockwise direction – down, forward, up and back – keep it as flowing movement rather than four positions. Have a visual image of large wheels turning backwards. Repeat twice.

iii) Rotate in an anti-clockwise direction – down, back, up and forward – in the same way and this time the large wheels turning forward. Repeat twice.

iv) Practise the clockwise and anti-clockwise movement with just the left shoulder up to four times, keeping the right shoulder quite still and relaxed.

Repeat with the right shoulder and keep the left shoulder still.

v) Repeat the first exercise by hunching the shoulders up *breathe in, hold the position and breath* for a moment – and *sigh deeply* as you drop the shoulders down – and let go.

vi) Complete these exercises by dropping the head forward and, with the fingers and palms of the hands, just pat the back of the neck and shoulders quickly and lightly and enjoy the tingling exhilarating effect when you stop.

3 Eyes

If you regularly wear spectacles and can feel safe without them please remove them for the following exercises:-

i) Blink the eyes in an exaggerated way – and let go. Having the eyes closed look to the left as though you can see inside your left ear, to the right as though you can see inside your right ear, look right up as though you can see inside the top of your head and down as though you can see inside your throat – and repeat once more.

ii) Still with the eyes closed rotate clockwise and then anti-clockwise twice each way.

Blink the eyes in an exaggerated way and then open them.

iii) Repeat the exercises with the eyes open. Keep the head quite still. If you have a tendency to move the head whilst moving the eyes then rest your finger tips of both hands lightly on the lower jaw to steady the head – this will encourage the eyes to work more. Look to the left, right, up and down. Repeat once more.

iv) Rotate the eyes in wide sweeping movements. Notice if and where the eyes have a tendency to laziness and blurred vision. Do not avoid these areas – on the contrary be very precise. Rotate up to three times each way. Blink the eyes in an exaggerated way – and relax.

Just check that you are not producing tension in the neck, throat, jaw or mouth whilst practising these exercises. Consciously disassociate other areas of the body. Swallow to release tension in the throat and check that the teeth are not clenched so releasing the jaw.

v) Exercise for the focussing muscles of the eyes.

Sit tall with eyes open and place your index finger in front of your eyes so that you can clearly see the tip. The proximity of the finger to your eyes will depend upon your eyesight – make the distance appropriate for you. Look from your finger to a point immediately beyond the finger and as far away as possible – with complete vision. Do this several times. Aim to have clear vision at each point before returning the gaze to the other point.

Blink the eyes in an exaggerated way and let go.

You can also practise this without using your finger when you are by the sea or out in the country where you have a good view to observe something very close by and very far away. For example, if by the sea, look from the mast of a boat nearby to a boat on the horizon. If you are in an area where you can see traffic a long way off trace one particular vehicle for as long as you can.

vi) Bring the palms of the hands together, rub them until they become quite warm and then place them over your closed eyes, and rest.

vii) Bring the three middle fingers of each hand to rest quite firmly over the eyes and exert a little pressure until you see *stars* – and let go.

Place the palms of the hands over the closed eyes again to rest them. Practising in this way you are utilising your natural warmth and life-force in the hands to enhance your eyes.

The eyes are such a sensitive and reflective area of the body. There is a fine dividing line between truly needing spectacles of varying strength and resorting to them through laziness and vanity. If you are on the borderline of requiring spectacles notice how, when you feel on top of the world and well, they do not seem to be so necessary – you may even forget about them. At this stage it is highlighted how the eyes reflect your state of general health and wellbeing.

Wearing sunglasses can become a habit which does not always do the eyes any favours. The eyes require light and air and when they are shielded behind dark lenses they are denied this natural resource. Obviously in very bright sun or snow it is essential to protect the eyes but overuse of sunglasses can be harmful.

Working and living in natural daylight is obviously preferable to artificial light, particularly fluorescent lighting which, over a period of time, can have a general debilitating effect.

Avoid overuse of eye drops unless under specific direction.

Additional exercises using the natural resource of sun and water

Sun exercise

Bathe the closed eyes in the morning sun. Sit for up to five minutes with sun playing on your closed eyelids. Turn the head to the left and let the sun shine on to the right temple and behind the eyes for up to a further five minutes and then turn the head to the right and repeat for a further five minutes. Then sit in the shade for a further five minutes and relax. Whilst practising in this way feel as though you are absorbing the sun's healing energy.

Water exercise

On rising in the morning splash the eyes well with cold water. You can bathe the eyes in plain water with an eye bath or fill a basin and lower your face into the water, open your eyes and rotate them two or three times each way.

Pat the face with a soft towel to remove excess water. Rub the palms of the hands well together and place them over your closed eyes for a few moments.

4 *Jaw*

The jaw has a powerful role to play in supporting the teeth to grind down food and chewing it in preparation for digestion. 'Grin and bear it' and 'Grit your teeth and think of the Motherland' are typical of the amount of energy that is put into holding back. Some people grind their teeth when listening to others whilst mulling or chewing over what is being said with an impatience to say their own piece. Grinding the teeth whilst sleeping could be a physical symptom of holding on or back from saying or shouting something and can lead to severe dental problems. Releasing tension from this area may well have a marked psychological as well as physical effect.

   i) Lie flat on the floor in order that the head is well supported with the back of the neck slightly stretched.

  ii) Open the mouth as wide as you can and stick the tongue out as far as you can. Hold that position for a moment – then withdraw the tongue and close the mouth without clenching the teeth. Repeat twice more.

 iii) Rotate the jaw slowly and thoroughly – clockwise four times and anti-clockwise four times.

 iv) Draw a figure of eight with your jaw. Repeat four times.

  v) Massage your jaw. Curl your forefingers round to form a hook shape, and, together with the thumbs massage the jaw on both sides – left side with left hand and right side with right hand. Using firm pressure start up by the ear and make small circular movements towards the chin until the forefingers meet. Then pinch the jaw between the forefingers and thumbs all the way back up to the ears in tine small movements.

Repeat twice more.

 vi) Finally just relax the whole face and check that the teeth are not clenched. Open your mouth as wide as possible and breathe in to the base of your throat and enjoy a sensuous y-a-w-n and relax.

5 *Fingers, hands and wrists*

Aim – to ease arthritis and tension in the hands and strengthen fingers and wrists.

a) i) Stand facing the wall at an arm's length away. Reach out to touch the wall with your fingers and place the palms of the hands flat on the wall.

ii) Keeping the palms in contact with the wall walk the hands upwards as far as you can. Aim to have a straight line from your heels to the tips of your fingers.

iii) Now walk the hands down in the same way. The weight of your body will help to ease your wrists.

Repeat twice more.

b) i) Sitting down bring the hands together in the prayer position – tips of the fingers, palms and heels of the hands touching.

ii) Splay the finger out into a fan shape keeping the same contact between the hands. Close them and repeat twice more.

iii) Interlace the fingers and turn the hands inside out with the palms facing outward straightening the arms away from you. Aim to have the thumbs and little fingers of each hand in close contact with each other. Ease the fingers out as much as you can.

iv) Release that hold – and return to the first position with palms of the hands together.

v) Interlace the fingers now in a different way. Probably the first time you did it it was a natural reaction for you to either bring the left thumb in front of the right – or vice versa. This time interlace the fingers so that the *other* thumb is in front and consequently the remaining fingers.

vi) Repeat the process by turning the hands inside out, palms and fingers away and straight arms. Hold that position.

vii) Release the hold and return to the first position.

6 Hand Massage
Use the hands to massage each other – first of all the left with the right

i) Begin by easing out the bed of the thumb nail.

ii) Take hold of the small joints of the thumb and knuckle and begin to unscrew them round and round.

iii) Finally hold the tip of the thumb and shake it vigorously. Repeat this process with each finger on the left hand.

iv) With pressure from the right thumb firmly push down between the left thumb and forefinger in small steps towards the wrist marking out the passage between the bone structure. Repeat this process between each finger. When you reach the outside of the little finger repeat in the same way just pinching the flesh with the thumb and forefinger of the right hand, until you reach the left wrist.

v) Turn the left hand uppermost and in the same way create pressure in the palm of the left hand with the right thumb in between the fingers and down to the wrist.

vi) Grasp the left wrist with the right hand and alternately make a screwing and unscrewing movement with the hand.

vii) Finally rub the palms of the hands together quite vigorously.

When you stop place the backs of the hands on your lap and experience the difference between the two hands. Repeat the whole process by massaging the right hand with the left and enjoy the tingling and comfortable effect in both hands.

9 Relax and Unwind

Relaxation Response and Rediscovery

Body and mind are capable of tremendous exertion and deep rest. There is natural ability to swing between the two as and when required and this state of wellbeing is known as homeostasis which is achieved through the balance of the autonomic nervous system and its two constituent parts of sympathetic and parasympathetic.

Just as there is a fight-or-flight response created by the sympathetic nervous system there is a relaxation response created by the parasympathetic nervous system. Unfortunately, the tendency in our fast moving society can be to place more emphasis on the activity of the sympathetic nervous system as this is the busy 'seen to be doing' attitude. The deeply passive state created by the action of the parasympathetic nervous system is there to balance. Ideally it comes naturally, but due to pressures and conditioning it has become a lost art and it is necessary to re-learn the *natural* skill. We need to know how to balance the highly active state with the deeply passive state and this can be learned with patience and diligence – simple but not necessarily easy.

Relaxation, like innocence, is there all the time – an integral part of ourselves. It is necessary to discover and re-discover this natural state.

The perfect antidote to stress

Tension builds up in muscles and if not released begins to *sit* in the body as though it is its right to be there. We then compound that by ignoring it and allowing it to accumulate. Tense shoulders, neck, jaw, hands, face, stomach, headache, backache, racing heart beat and indigestion are just the beginning!

Exhaustion and tiredness eventually lead to inefficiency. 'Prevention is better than cure' is an old adage which may well be true in this case. Learning a simple skill to elicit and evoke the relaxation response can balance the whole system and render it more efficient.

Although relaxation is an obvious and perfect antidote to stress it may well be that prevention is *not* always better than cure as, for some people, it is necessary to experience the depth of despair and pain – driven to the nth degree of physical, mental, emotional trauma before changing and even then it may still be the choice not to change.

However, relaxation is a gentle art that allows you to be in charge of yourself all the time – no manipulation, no cutting off the senses, no brainwashing – just a simple clearing of the mind to produce a deep state of restful alertness that rejuvenates and normalises the function of the central nervous system. It could be termed 'mental hygiene'. Inner wisdom is developed so that unprogrammed learning takes place beyond expectation.

When we release our narrowed blinkered view of just wishing to overcome distress, disability or disease we leave ourselves open to experience the hitherto *unexperienced* and this is how learning takes place with development, expansion and inreading awareness of what is about us.

The five senses play their part in the physical world. The sixth sense of intuition is developed in deep relaxation – 'in'tuition – a knowing from within – that innate wisdom. It is our true nature to be highly creative but we naively place limitations upon ourselves through a lack of trust.

Physiological changes

The physiological changes of the relaxation responses are in direct opposition to those changes that are noted in the fight-or-flight response:-

FIGHT OR FLIGHT RESPONSE	RELAXATION RESPONSE
produced by activity of	produced by activity of
sympathetic nervous system	parasympathetic nervous system

Increased	Decreased
Heart rate	
Blood pressure	
Breathing rate	
Oxygen consumption	
Carbon dioxide elimination	
Metabolic rate	
Muscle tension	
Blood lactate level★	
Blood flow to extremities	

★Anxiety is associated with high levels of lactate which is a substance produced by skeletal muscles and, when in tension, traps the oxygen within muscles.

Brain waves

The brain has two hemispheres with a connective tissue known as the corpus callosum, body of fibres, about one inch deep. These two cerebral hemispheres have two quite separate functions:

Left hemisphere is associated with	Right hemisphere is associated with
speech	intuition
logic	body image
language	creativity
questions	emotional appreciation
analysis	3D imaging
mathematics	feeling
crossword sequence	art
clock time	left-handedness
deduction	

The Western education system encourages dominance of the left hemisphere.

Brain wave patterns are measurable by electroencephalograph. In normal everyday existence one hemisphere has dominance over the other at any given time depending upon the mode and mood of the moment, the attitude and personality. Ideally they alternate and respond to each other. In deep relaxation, meditation and highly creative ecstatic states it is shown that both sides of the brain are functioning equally giving enhanced perception. This pattern has also been found in small children deeply immersed in play.

The rhythm of the nerve current is measured in cycles per second (cps) and there are four main patterns indicated:

Associated with

Delta waves 0 – 4 cps	deep sleep
Theta waves 4 – 7 cps	creativity, flash of insight, creative problem solving, dreaming, vision, inner consciousness of sleep, painless surgery
Alpha waves 7 – 14 cps	emotional tranquillity, relaxed state of mind, day dreaming, extra-sensory perception, meditation, self-healing
Beta waves 14 plus cps	waking state reflecting the outside world through the five senses

It is the *alpha* and *theta* waves that are associated with deep relaxation, meditation, creativity and emotional tranquillity.

Attention without tension

Observing animals can teach us a lot about relaxed living and conserving energy. Watch them as they enquire, convey a message, stalk, listen, sense, stretch, rest and sleep. They have the natural ability to be totally alert when required and deeply relaxed when not, but still with restful awareness. We too have that natural ability but due to civilisation, conditioning, expectation and losing touch with the natural rhythm within and around us it can become a lost art. We need to be skilled to live and live well – and this has very little to do with material wealth.

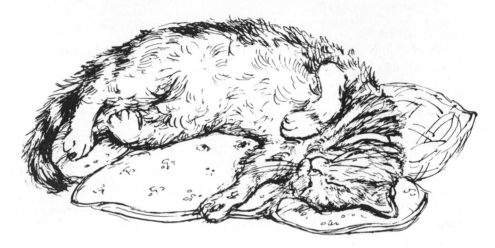

The release of tension is a personal choice. It is up to *you*. Faulty physical, mental and emotional habits that go unrecognised or ignored can build from a niggling tension to real discomfort and 'dis'ease. However, the solace is that if it is *you* that has created the situation it is also *you* who can change it.

Communication between mind and body can lead to a deeper understanding of ourselves and our own true nature. Through *minding your body* you can begin to release unwanted tension, adjust to stress and guide the imagination to a state of high level *wellness*. Relaxation is a natural state and needs to be rediscovered. However, it is not just stopping to have a cup of coffee, to sit in front of the television, lie down and listen to music or fall asleep. All of these can be very restful pursuits but in learning and developing these new skills there is a conscious decision made to become aware of tension and relaxation and for the mind to focus attention on one specific thing at a time. In concentration and controlling thought at will it is possible to reach a point of stillness that resides within, the point of stillness that is masked by the constant activity of the mind. Through relaxing in this way you can begin to *let go*, release unnecessary tension, accept or change difficult situations, adjust attitudes and move towards achieving a balanced state of equilibrium.

The sense of stillness can give rise to creativity and it *is* creative because *you* are doing it. Relaxation is not necessarily an end in itself but more a tool for releasing unwanted physical, mental and emotional tensions and anxieties. It could be likened to passing through a doorway to a new way of living.

Personal observations

After practising relaxation for a while people generally notice an enhanced sense of well-being and often find a new avenue of interest previously unexplored, social ease, confidence, more warmth and enjoyment between family, friends and creative expression. The process of simply *letting go* can release previously blocked energy which can then be channelled creatively and this can result in creative problem solving too.

The following is just an example of the many verbal comments and letters received from people who have attended relaxation courses and/or used the cassette tapes on relaxation:

'I now have more energy to enjoy my life'

'I am really grateful to that stressful time and learning about relaxation as it has taught me so much about myself and life that I might never have known'

'Even though I am physically limited as a result of the cardiac arrest I can truly say that I now have an inner fulfilment'

'No longer do I have to dominate a situation or people in order to feel safe, as relaxation has helped me to develop my own self-confidence'

'Please let this information help other people with neck and shoulder tension – I used to spend a lot of money each month getting my tight neck and shoulders pummelled out, but now, through a relaxed body and mind, the tension is virtually non-existent'

'I no longer dread going to bed as sleep comes easily to me now'

'I have started to paint landscapes – something I have wanted to do since I was a child'

'In taking responsibility for myself I now appreciate other people far more'

. . . and so on.

It is generally the *need* to relax that attracts people to seek out these hidden jewels that lead to so much. It is the headaches, high blood pressure, asthma, insomnia, fear, anxiety, panic attacks, over smoking, over drinking, tranquillisers, stomach upsets etc. that eventually drive towards self improvement.

When anxious or upset it is not unusual to be told 'Go away and learn to relax', 'calm down', 'cool it', but in order for relaxation skills to be effective it is necessary for them to be established well and this requires diligent practice which is the groundwork that reaps best results. The natural state of relaxation achieved by oneself then surely becomes preventive medicine at its best.

Relaxed living

These simple techniques are recommended by doctors, therapists and healers to create the most conducive internal environment for true healing to take place. In fact, once the environment has been created and a genuine gesture is made towards *real health* Nature seems to take over. Often this is all that is required to restore the balance.

The success of the exercise depends entirely upon and you and your commitment and attitude. The only requirements from you are a decision to positively choose to learn to relax and a commitment of regular practice at a habit-forming time.

Treat this as a training programme in order to learn a new skill. Do not have preconceived ideas as these can be limiting – just remain open and receptive. You will be setting out on a journey which can lead to changes in your lifestyle and attitude. Relaxation will help you take this journey – it just requires commitment to practice. It is not necessary for you to set about making difficult changes in your life or doing without the things that you enjoy. Once you begin to practise these simple exercises on a regular basis you will find that changes may occur naturally for your own benefit. Although you may only practise for ten minutes once or twice a day this will affect the remaining 23 hours and 50 minutes, and enhance the quality of your life. This is not about cutting down an external stress – although that can happen – it is more about learning to adjust.

Advantages of learning and practising the simple relaxation skills are many, highly individual, and include the following:

- heighten the awareness of *hidden* physical and mental tension
- ease and release tense nerves, muscles and psychosomatic tension and pain
- improve appearance through releasing strain and tension
- improve general physical health and strengthen the immune system
- produce more energy and vitality by releasing tension
- improve quality of sleep
- improve self-image and self-confidence
- get to know oneself better, to become more creative and realise potential
- to become more at one, in tune and at peace with oneself
- become more effective and relaxed for oneself and others
- decrease emotional disturbance and need for stimulants, smoking, alcohol, drugs, tranquillisers and anti-depressants

. . . and more . . .

General suggestions

Avoid using the time to opt out by sleeping or working things out through logical thought. Sometimes it is absolutely inevitable that sleep comes, perhaps this is what is most needed at the time. Enormous benefit can be gained from remaining totally awake and aware and truly focusing the attention. Allow relaxation to lead you to become aware of your inner self and let that awareness lead you to harmony between physical body, mental attitude, emotional stability and spiritual wellbeing.

You may find that really good ideas come to you either during or after relaxation – observe them as they may well be relevant to your present situation. Catch the thoughts and ideas at their conception and follow them as they could lead you to enjoy fresh experience, to become 'as a little child' in sheer enjoyment of experience. You may like to keep a pencil and pad beside you so that you can write down these ideas after the relaxation as reminders. However, avoid using the time to plan through logical thought.

Environment

The ideal place for you to practise this exercise is a warm, draught-free pleasant place where you can be quiet and without interruption. If necessary put a 'Please do not disturb' notice on the door and take the telephone off the hook. If you feel it is appropriate inform the people who are close to you of your intention – this can help to establish your commitment and may well give you support and encouragement.

Create a habit in time and place. First thing in the morning just after you wake up helps set the tone for the day. Times of natural break e.g. mid-morning, mid-afternoon or early evening suit some people, and last thing at night can lead to a good night's sleep.

Clothing You do not want to be bothered with tight restricting clothes so loosen anything that is tight like collar, tie or belt and slip off your shoes.

Regularity is of utmost importance. Practise once a day if you can at least four times a week. Obviously the more you practise efficiently the greater accumulative effect you will experience. Once you have established a regular pattern and have become familiar with the technique you will then be able to practise it at other times and in other places.

The techniques in this section are written in such a way that you can practise with another person – partner, loved one or friend. Help yourselves as you take turns to read through the script to one another. In this way you will quickly learn the sequence and then be able to practise quietly on your own.

I   *Relax and unwind*

II *Body awareness and conscious disassociation*

III *Trio:*

   a) Neuro-muscular relaxation

   b) Complete deep relaxation – and in prone position

   c) Solar breathing

IV *Imagination and visualisation*

i RELAX AND UNWIND

A brief, practical technique using key words as suggestions. The aims are not modest:

- consciously release tension in body, mind and emotions
- elicit the relaxation response

- restore energy
- release negative thought patterns
- tap into your own stillness within
- prepare a new environment for creative living
- enjoy a natural break.

   i) Sit in the Basic Sitting Position. In order to use the recall technique referred to later take up the following hand position: Place the pads of the forefingers against the pads of the thumbs on each hand.

   ii) Close your eyes and begin to withdraw the attention from the external world. Become aware of *how you feel physically* this very moment. Notice where you feel comfortable, uncomfortable or not necessarily anything . . . then release the attention to that.

   iii) Become aware of your *thoughts* – what is uppermost in your mind. Observe your thoughts as things and be prepared to mentally watch them. Follow those thoughts – and let them go at will. Just be prepared to put them to one side – at least for the next few minutes.

   iv) Bring your attention to *here and now* – this very moment. Consciously release all that is past, even just a moment ago. Release all that has yet to come and all that is elsewhere present. Simply say to yourself . . . 'I am preparing to relax . . . I am preparing to relax'. Devote your total attention to the statement.

   v) *Allow* your eyelids and forehead to feel smooth. Begin to relax from the top of your head down – inside your head, your eyes, all parts of your face, feeling smooth and calm. Check that your teeth are not clenched so releasing the jaw. Swallow to release any tension that may have gathered in your throat. Relax into the back of your neck, shoulders, arms and hands. Become aware of your back, its shape and slight curve into the back of your waist – and let go. Feel your body softening. Become aware of your chest cavity, housing your heart and lungs – and relax that area deeply. Soften into the solar plexus and deep into the abdomen. Relax your legs and feet.

   vi) To deepen concentration incline your closed eyes up as though you are looking inside and behind the forehead – above and between the eyebrows.

   vii) Without changing its pattern just recognise the fact that you are breathing . . . Notice your breath . . . Avoid trying to do anything other than observe the breath.

The breath is happening – just as it always has happened although it may now have become quite shallow and gentle. Just *allow the breath to happen*. Play the role of the silent witness of the breath . . . After a short while you may experience a slight shift of atmosphere so that it is not so much that you are breathing but that *you are being breathed*.

You are at the *end* of the breath.

You are as much a part of the breath as the breath is a part of you.

viii) Begin to notice the two main parts of the breath – inhalation and exhalation.

As you breathe in run the attention from the base of the spine to the top of the head.
As you breathe out run the attention down over the front of the body.
Continue to do this entirely in your own time.
Breathe in – bring the attention from the base of the spine to the top of your head checking your upright and comfortable posture.
Breathe out – run the attention down over the front of your body without slumping.

ix) Gradually allow the exhalation to become a little longer. Recognise that this is the part of the breath that is constantly releasing, relaxing and letting go. Tune into these natural qualities – releasing, relaxing and letting go . . .

x) After a while you may notice the other two parts of the breath. There is a momentary pause between the inhalation and exhalation and another between the exhalation and inhalation.

Focus the attention in particular on the pause *after* the exhalation.

xi) At the every end of that pause simply say to yourself . . . relax . . . relax . . . Repeat that simple suggestion to yourself each time you reach the end of the pause after the exhalation. Repeat it until you *feel* relaxation flowing and glowing within. Let that develop. At the next pause at the end of the exhalation say to yourself . . . let go . . . let go . . . Repeat this to yourself as you *feel* all unnecessary tensions just leaving you – all physical, mental and emotional tension just *leaving*. Let go . . . *feel* it happening . . .

xii) Keep your attention on the end of the pause after each exhalation and develop the suggestion as you say to yourself be still . . . be still . . . be still . . . and then just be . . . Remain in that stillness for a few minutes. Gradually you will begin to develop contact with that which resides deep within you.

xiii) From that point of stillness bring the attention slowly back to the gentle natural rhythmic flow of the inhalation and exhalation. Let the breath deepen a little and as you breathe in bring the attention up through the front of the body feeling the chest open and comfortable. As you breathe out run the attention down over your back. Repeat this several times and, as the saying goes, 'like water off a duck's back'. Feel almost as though your feathers are being smoothed down. Remind yourself of the experience of focusing your attention on the breath and your key words.

Relax . . . Let go . . . Be still . . . Be
Recognise and remember the value of the experience so that you can recall it at other times.

xiv) Decide when you are going to practise this exercise again and make the commitment to yourself *now*. Become aware of *here and now* this very moment and where you are. Listen to any sounds, and remind yourself of the time of day and what you will be doing next.

xv) Prepare to stretch and move as you bring the palms of your hands together, rub them, and place them over your eyes. Have a really good s-t-r-e-t-c-h, release your hands and look around you at your familiar surroundings again.

Take that feeling of relaxation with you and enjoy the recharging effect that restful awareness can bring.

With regular practice, this simple technique will be affecting every cell in your body, every part of your mind and emotions – your whole wellbeing.

Recall

The physical body has a memory and stores experience in the flesh. Imitating a position, movement or gesture can remind the body and mind of that experience.

The groundwork of regular practice must be done first. Once you have experienced the state of deep relaxation you will be able to recall that state at other times to suit you. For example –

- when you need to collect your thoughts and review what has gone on before
- when you feel tired or anxious in order to calm down and revive yourself
- before meetings and starting new projects
- before interviews and exams etc.
- at times when you need to have your wits about you – being alert yet calm and collected. This could help you to see things objectively rather than becoming caught up and taken over by the situation.
- a highly charged emotional situation or when everything is crowding in and at times of panic.

Practise the art of recall

Remind yourself of the state of deep restfulness by imitating the body language and physical gesture that you made whilst deeply relaxing.

It need not be obvious to anyone else as you shift your posture in a very subtle way.

  i) Exhale – let go first of all.
 ii) Take a deep quiet breath into the base of the lungs, lengthen the spinal column, open out your chest without necessarily moving your arms, place the fingers together as in the optional recommended gesture and remind yourself of the quiet restful state that you achieved.
iii) Exhale – relax and let go whilst you maintain the body shape and gesture.
iv) Concentrate totally on the breath as you continue to breathe evenly, gently and deeply into the base of the lungs and exhale by drawing in the abdomen. Repeat several times until the hiatus subsides.

The recall process is at its most efficient when you have established the groundwork well.

ii BODY AWARENESS AND CONSCIOUS DISASSOCIATION

Aims to:

- highlight tension of which you may already be aware and let it go
- discover hidden tension, become aware of it and let it go
- experience the effect that tension and relaxation has upon the breath
- experience the difference between tense and relaxed muscles
- become aware of the body mimicking itself
- learn the art of holding certain parts of the body in tension when required and releasing others when not required
- gain control over tight tense muscles
- enjoy a deep physical relaxation.

The order in which to tighten and relax the body is as follows:

1 Lower – from feet to waist

2 Left leg

3 Right leg

4 Upper – from fingers and waist to head

5 Left arm

6 Right arm

7 Left side

8 Right side

9 Left arm to right leg

10 Right arm to left leg

11 Review

12 Deeply relax and let go.

Conscious disassociation

Lie flat on the floor (see Appendix) and allow yourself to relax from the top of your head to the tips of your toes.

1) a) Take your attention to your feet, tighten up the muscles in the lower part of your body by pushing your heels away, open out your toes, tighten the calf muscles, knees, thigh muscles, groin and buttocks and draw in the perineum as though you are trying to stop yourself from releasing urine or having a bowel movement. Draw the abdomen in tight as though you are trying to get into a pair of trousers one size too small. Hold all this tension very very tight and *become aware of what tight tense muscles feel like* in the lower part of your body.

LIVERPOOL
JOHN MOORES UNIVERSITY
AVRIL ROBARTS LRC
TEL. 0151 231 4022

b) Whilst holding that tension, consciously disassociate other parts of the body that are not required in tension at the moment. Relax your chest and back, your hands from the tips of your fingers, palms of the hands, wrists, lower arms, upper arms and shoulders. Swallow to release any tension in the throat. Soften in the back of the neck and base of the skull, check that your teeth are not clenched so relaxing the jaw. Relax all the tiny little muscles in the face, particularly around the eyes and brow – and now the very top of your head. Notice any tendency to hold on to tension in specific parts of your upper body – notice this for future reference.

Notice that *you* have consciously disassociated the lower part of your body in tension from the upper part which is relaxed.

c) Breathe in, tighten the lower part of your body just a little more and as you sigh deeply out of the mouth completely let go from the waist down, abdomen, buttocks, groin, thighs, knees, calves, ankles, insteps and toes. Feel tension draining out of the body long after the end of the deep sigh. Keep letting go . . . and enjoy relaxed muscles in the lower part of your body.

2) a) Repeat this exercise with just the left leg. Push the heel away, open out your toes, tighten the calf muscles, knee and thigh and left buttock.

b) As you hold that tension consciously disassociate the right foot, leg, buttock and let the right leg be loose and floppy. Relax all other parts of the body that you do not need to hold in tension at this time – back, abdomen, chest, fingers, hands, arms, shoulders, throat, neck, face and head. Notice any tendency to hold the breath and aim to breathe naturally. Notice any tendency to hold tension in specific areas. Observe how *you* have consciously disassociated the tense left leg from the loose right leg and other parts of your body.

c) Breathe in and tighten your left leg a little more and, as you sigh deeply, completely let go from the left buttock, thigh, knee, calf and foot. Feel tension draining out of the left leg long after the end of the exhalation and – let go.

Keep letting go. Notice the different feeling between the left leg that has been tense and the right leg that has been relaxed.

3) Repeat this exercise by tightening the right leg and keeping the left leg loose and floppy, relaxing the remainder of the body.

4) Bring your attention to your hands, arms and shoulders.

a) Raise your arms upwards and open out your fingers as wide as you can. Tighten the muscles in your shoulders, back and chest as you reach up high. Keeping your eyes closed screw your face up as tight as you can and raise your head, neck and shoulders off the floor and really stretch up – and hold tight.

b) Whilst holding that tension consciously disassociate the lower part of your body – hips, buttocks, legs and feet – let it all be very relaxed. Notice the tendency to hold the breath and specific parts of the body that are not required at this stage. Notice how tense muscles feel.

c) Breathe in a little deeper, increase the tension and then, as you sigh deeply – let go and carefully lower your head, arms and hands to the floor. Relax from the top of your head and all parts of your face – eyes, mouth, jaw; swallow to release the throat, relax the back of the neck, shoulders, arms and hands. Relax deeply into the chest and back and down into your abdomen, buttocks, legs and feet. Really experience the difference between tight and relaxed muscles in the top part of your body.

5) Bring your attention to the left hand, arm and shoulder.

a) Raise your left arm off the floor, open your fingers out as wide as you can, stretch up and tighten the muscles in your left shoulder.

Notice how it all feels.

b) Whilst holding tension in the left arm and shoulder consciously disassociate the muscles in your face, jaw, neck, throat, right shoulder, arm and hand and relax them. Soften in the back, deep into the chest, abdomen, groin and legs. Notice any tendency to hold the breath and aim to breathe naturally. Notice any tendency to hold particular parts of your body in tension that are not required at this time.

c) Breathe in a little deeper, tighten the muscles in the left arm and shoulder a little more and then as you sigh deeply lower the arm to the floor and completely let go.

Relax from the top of the head down into both shoulders, arms and hands, the back, chest, abdomen, buttocks, legs and feet. Notice how the muscles feel in your left shoulder, arm and hand.

6) Repeat this exercise by tightening the right arm and shoulder.

7) Bring your attention to the left side of your body from the tips of your toes to the tips of your fingers.

a) Push the heel of your left foot away and open out your toes. Tighten up the calf, knee, thigh and left buttock. Raise your left arm up and behind your head so that the back of the hand touches the floor. Open out your fingers and really s-t-r-e-t-c-h your left heel and left hand away. Open out the left side of your ribcage and s-t-r-e-t-c-h.

b) Notice the tendency for the right side to join in. Consciously disassociate as you relax in the forehead, eyes, jaws, right shoulder and arm, chest, abdomen, right buttock and foot. Notice any tendency to hold the breath and aim to breathe naturally.

c) Breathe in a little more deeply as you stretch a little further. Hold the stretch and then, as you sigh deeply, bring the left arm back by your side and completely let go.

Notice the difference between the left side of the body that has been stretched and the right side.

8) Repeat this exercise by tightening up the right side of the body.

9) Bring your attention to your left arm and right leg as you create a diagonal stretch.

a) Raise your left arm up and over your head, back of the hand on the floor and open out the fingers wide. Push your right heel away and open out the toes. Create a long diagonal stretch across from the heel on the right foot and the fingers on the left hand.

b) As you hold that stretch consciously disassociate other parts of the body – jaw, face, back of the neck, right shoulder, arm and hand, left leg and foot. Notice any tendency to hold the breath and aim to breathe naturally. Notice any tendency to consistently produce tension in other parts of the body.

c) Breathe in, stretch a little further and, as you lower the left arm back by your side, sigh deeply out of the mouth.

Experience the relaxed muscles of your left arm and right leg in particular.

10) Repeat this exercise by raising the right arm up and back and pushing the left heel away. Notice any real difference between left and right sides of your body.

11) As you rest just review the experience.

i) Remind yourself of any particular areas of your body that consistently become tense when not required to be so. Keep this information for your future reference and make a conscious decision to periodically check this area of the body throughout the day. If you notice that it has become tense then tighten it up a little more and really exaggerate it beyond its habitual tense state. Breathe in and hold on to that tension for a moment and then, as you sigh deeply out of the mouth, completely let go. Repeat this twice more.

ii) Remind yourself of any tendency to hold the breath whilst producing tension. In the same way periodically check your breathing throughout the day particularly when you are concentrating and if you catch yourself holding your breath then just stop what you are doing for a moment and let it go. Breathe deeply and gently and, when you have re-established an easy rhythm, continue with what you were doing.

12) Finally – push your heels away, tighten up your legs, buttocks, abdomen, back and chest. Open your fingers wide and tighten up the muscles of your arms and shoulders. Raise the head, neck and shoulders off the floor as you screw your face up tight. Hold that tension for a moment and then, as you sigh deeply, completely let go beyond the end of the exhalation and allow yourself to soften and relax into the floor – releasing, relaxing and letting go.

iii TRIO

a) Neuro–muscular relaxation

b) Complete deep relaxation – and in prone position

c) Solar breathing

These three exercises *naturally follow each other* but *it is not necessary to do all three every time.*

i) Learn the technique of neuro–muscular relaxation and periodically check yourself throughout the day as suggested.

ii) Learn the complete deep relaxation – this is the one to aim to practise every day, with or without the others. It is also the one that is suggested at the end of the physical exercise programmes.

Try lying prone as an alternative some time – you may discover other benefits.

iii) Learn to use your creative imagination and develop the solar breathing.

If you prefer to work with relaxation on cassette you will find these three together on *Relax Your Mind and Body*.

iiia) **Neuro-muscular relaxation**

Aims to:

● increase awareness of tension and relaxation in various parts of the body
● exercise control over excess tension
● deeply relax.

This form of relaxation exercise involves systematically tightening and relaxing muscles from the tips of the toes to the top of the head. Each time you tighten the muscles notice the resulting tension and as you relax them experience the difference.

In the following order

1 Basic Lying or Sitting Position

2 Left foot, calf, knee, thigh

3 Right foot, calf, knee, thigh

4 Abdomen, buttocks, perineum

5 Chest and upper back

6 Left hand, fingers, wrist, fore arm, elbow, upper arm and left shoulder

7 Right hand, fingers, wrist, fore arm, elbow, upper arm and right shoulder

8 Face and head – jaw, tongue, mouth, eyes, throat, back of the neck, base of the skull

9 Relaxation without movement.

1 Take up the Basic Lying Position. Settle into a restful mode and, as you notice the breath, focus on relaxing more and more deeply with each exhalation.

2 i) Bring your attention to the left foot. Push your heel away hard then point your toes; then push the heel away again. Rotate the foot and ankle twice each way. Just wriggle the toes around and loosen the foot before really letting go.

ii) Tighten up the calf, knee and thigh whilst keeping the foot as relaxed as you can. Let it go.

iii) Tighten up the whole leg – push the heel away, flex the calf, knee and thigh. Hold that very tight . . . and let go completely.

3 Repeat with the right foot and leg.

4 Pull your abdomen in very tight and draw in your buttocks and the floor of the perineum. Keep the legs loose. Hold the tension . . . and let go.

5 Tighten up the muscles of the chest and upper back – hold that very tight. You may well recognise this as the kind of action you make when you are either very cold or frightened. Tightening in this way restricts the blood flow and is working against free circulation and warmth – just notice how we work against ourselves sometimes and the next time you catch yourself doing this consciously aim to relax.

6 i) Bring your attention to the left hand and fingers. Open out the fingers wide as though you are trying to reach beyond an octave on the piano; clench the fist tight – then open the fingers wide again. Rotate the hand and wrist twice each way. Wriggle the fingers around a little and let the hand be loose, and let go.

   ii) Tighten up the fore arm, elbow, upper arm and left shoulder whilst keeping the hand quite loose. Hold that tight – and let go.

   iii) Raise the arm off the floor, open the fingers wide, tighten up the fore arm, elbow, upper arm and left shoulder. Hold that very very tight . . . and let go.

7 Repeat with the right hand and arm.

8 i) Clench the teeth to tighten the jaw and push the tongue up against the roof of the mouth.

   ii) Keeping the teeth together part the lips to bare your teeth like a Cheshire cat. Then purse the lips together very tight.

   iii) Screw the eyes up tight and create furrows in your brow.

   iv) Tighten up the throat, back of the neck and base of the skull. Do you recognise any of this tension? Become very familiar with how this feels and recognise fully that these muscles are in tension through conscious choice . . . and completely let go.

9 Bring all that together by tightening up the jaw, lips, eyes, brow, throat and back of the neck as before. Hold on to that tension and raise your head, neck and shoulders . . . hold tight for a moment . . . and completely let go.

10 From the very beginning now to combine all areas –

   i) push your heels away and tighten up calves, knees and thighs

   ii) pull your abdomen in and tighten your buttocks and groin

   iii) tighten up your chest and back

   iv) open your fingers out wide and raise your arms as high as you can and hold in full tension.

   v) Screw the face up tight and raise your head, neck and shoulders.

   vi) Hold all that tension and the breath . . . and completely let go. During the day periodically check your body for tension when sitting, standing or lying down. In practising this exercise you will increase your awareness of tension in your muscles. The exercise is one of *consciously* choosing to create tension in the muscles in order to experience it. During the day at other times you may well find that you have *unconsciously* created tension in your muscles. Through the neuro-muscular relaxation exercise you will then recognise it more easily and can *consciously choose* to let it go at will – therefore releasing tension before it has a chance to accumulate into something more than just muscle tension. Notice tension in other people too – this will help you to learn more about yourself. Observation is a great teacher and a great way of putting the information into practice.

If you choose to bring your relaxation to a close at this point instead of continuing with the Complete Deep Relaxation please pay particular attention to the way in which you get up from the floor. (See Appendix 'Getting up from the floor.)

iiib) Complete deep relaxation

Complements the neuro-muscular relaxation and is very effective on its own particularly after physical exercise.
Aims to:

- Release physical and mental tension.
- Deeply relax body and mind and encourage an increased awareness of the effect that they have upon each other.
- Develop the creative imagination and powers of visualisation.

1 Basic Lying Position

2 Left foot and leg

3 Right foot and leg

4 Spinal column and back

5 Groin, abdomen, solar plexus

6 Chest cavity – heart and lungs

7 Left hand and arm

8 Right hand and arm

9 Throat, neck

10 Face – jaw, mouth, eyes and forehead, and all parts of the head

11 Visualise and relax.

1 Take up the Basic Lying Position.

2 Focus attention on the left leg and visualise each toe. Relax from the tip of each toe into the foot, the sole of the foot, instep, top of the foot, heel and ankle. Visualise the whole foot relaxed – and let go. Visualise the whole length of your leg and relax the

calf muscles, around the knee and thigh muscles. Feel the whole length of the left leg warm and tingly – and let go.

3 Repeat with the right foot and leg.

Both feet and legs now really relaxed, warm and tingly.

4 Visualise your spinal column supple and strong and relax from the base of the spine into the back of your waist, between the shoulder blades and back of the neck. Although the lumbar spine may not touch the floor allow it to sink down into the floor – really softening – and let go.

Feel that warmth and relaxation radiating out to the sides of your back enveloping you like a warm blanket.

5 Visualise your groin, abdomen and solar plexus soft, and glowing with health – and relax deeply.

6 Take your attention to your chest cavity housing your heart and lungs.

Visualise the heart and lungs communicating and working together perfectly to produce efficient circulation throughout all parts of your body. Relax deeply as you visualise that happening – and let go.

7   i) Take your attention to your left hand and visualise each finger. Relax from the tip of each finger into the hand. Relax the palm of the hand, back of the hand and wrist and visualise the whole hand soft and relaxed – and let go.

    ii) Visualise your fore arm, elbow, upper arm and left shoulder – relax – and let go.

8 Repeat with the right hand, arm and shoulder. Both hands, arms and shoulders now thoroughly relaxed, warm and tingly.

9 Swallow to release any tension that may have gathered in your throat and let go.

Relax into the back of the neck and base of the skull – consciously relax this area – and let go.

10 Check that the teeth are not clenched so releasing the jaw and relax all the tiny little muscles around the mouth, inside the mouth, cheeks, temples, and ears.

Relax the eyes, eyelids and forehead. Visualise your whole face smooth, relaxed and glowing with health. Relax the very top of your head and inside your head – and let go.

11 Visualise your whole body supple, strong and glowing with vibrant health and allow yourself to relax more and more deeply for a few more minutes.

If you intend getting up at this point instead of practising the Solar Breathing please remember to take care. (see Appendix, Getting up from the floor.)

Complete deep relaxation – lying prone

The compression of the chest and abdomen against the floor helps to encourage air into the sides and back of the lungs, eases digestion and flattens the abdomen.

1 Lie prone – flat on the floor with face down. Either rest the forehead on the backs of the hands or have the side of the face on the floor, changing to the other side of the face part way through the relaxation – this will help to ease the back of the neck and shoulder muscles.

2 Have your legs away from each other with feet turned in comfortably.

3 Arms resting on the floor around and above the head.

4 Deeply rest into the floor – toes, feet, legs, whole length of the back. Relax the groin, abdomen and chest just sinking into the floor. Relax the shoulders, arms and hands, the back of the neck and deep into the head and face.

5 Breathe easily, deeply and naturally and become aware of the compression that has been created in the chest by lying in this way. Notice how, *as you breathe in, the air is encouraged into the sides and back of the lungs.* Accentuate it slightly for a few breaths and feel the expansion in that area, and then relax deeply, breathing naturally. Become sensitive to the force of gravity at play. Visualise little arrows pinning you to the floor as you sink more and more deeply into relaxation.

Rest and relax concentrating on expansion in the sides and back of the lungs.

   After a few minutes begin to stretch your arms in front of you and prepare to leave that state as you open your eyes. Place your hands beside your shoulders and prepare to raise the head, neck and shoulders and come up on to the knees, and up to sitting position.

iiic) Solar breathing

Aim to:

- develop your creative imagination and visualisation

- create a receptive internal environment so that the body and mind can realise their full potential to heal themselves. Most benefit can be gained by first practising the Complete Deep Relaxation through the second part of this trio. Attention should be given to the following order:

1 Basic Lying Position

2 Beyond the top of your head

3 All parts of your body

4 Particular parts of the body that cause discomfort

5 Solar plexus

6 All parts of your body.

1 Basic Lying Position.

2 Using your creative imagination visualise a ball of energy – your own personal sunshine, immediately above and beyond the top of your head. Visualise that sunshine full of warmth and comfort radiating its healing rays.

3 Hold that powerful visual image and allow the warmth to permeate through into the very top of your head, into all parts of your face, throat, neck, shoulders, arms and hands, deep into your chest, solar plexus, abdomen, the whole length of your back and deep into your groin, legs and feet. Experience your whole body bathed in golden light and glowing with warmth.

4 If there is a particular part of your body that causes discomfort then *draw* golden light and warmth into that area. Hold it there and, in your imagination, visualise and feel the golden warmth glowing and melting away any discomfort. If it helps to establish the area then create physical contact by bringing the palms of the hands to rest on the area. Allow the healing energy to flow.

5 To create a general boost of energy focus the attention on your solar plexus – just above the navel and below the rib cage. Bring your hands to rest there and experience this area as a powerhouse of energy pulsating and glowing with vibrant health.

6 Allow that energy from your solar plexus to radiate out to all parts of your body – into your back, down into the abdomen, legs and feet; up into your chest, shoulders, arms and hands; into the throat, neck, face and head. Experience that glowing warmth in all parts of your body and visualise yourself glowing with vibrant health. Take care in getting up from the floor.

iv IMAGINATION AND VISUALISATION

The imagination is immensely powerful and responsible for everything you do. Visualisation uses the imagination to create what you want in your life – to sense and feel without physically seeing. The way that you perceive yourself is the way that you are. If you have a good self-image you create just that. Conversely if you have a bad self-image you create that too. You can limit and expand your potential within the imagination. You attract and repel situations and people to yourself as a result of your imagination.

To be aware of the power of the imagination and visualisation can be the key to making decisions about what to visualise in order to create what you truly want.

If you constantly think of illness you begin to have an illness consciousness that is thinking in terms of illness and is directly opposed to thinking in terms of wellness. You are therefore most likely to become ill rather than well. The more positive energy you radiate the more you will attract. Being fearful, anxious and afraid may well attract the very situation and people that you are trying to avoid. In no way is this a suggestion that you ignore being fearful, anxious and afraid pretending that the danger is not there. It is a suggestion to dwell more upon the positive aspect.

Energy follows thought

Create a visual image of something that you do not like – a situation in which you feel anxious, threatened or afraid. Close your eyes for a moment as you visualise yourself in that situation. Notice how you feel physically and mentally – are there changes in your breathing rate, heart beat, shoulders, neck, stomach? Has it reminded you of something unpleasant? – Notice your thoughts.

Now create a visual image of something that you like – a situation in which you feel comfortable, confident and happy. Close your eyes for a moment as you visualise yourself in that situation. Notice how you feel and how your thoughts have developed.

Have you noticed any difference between the two reactions? If you did it effectively you will most probably have noticed that your imagination, visualisation and thought reached your feelings and your body. This is precisely the pattern that creates body changes to display degrees of illness and wellness.

Energy follows thought. When you begin to practise and believe that you can go from strength to strength.

Create your own visual image

To use this in a creative way you can create a pleasing visual image of a place where you like to be – a place that gives you a sense of safety, security, comfort, joy and wellbeing. It may be anywhere that is already familiar to you – like a beautiful garden, woodland walk, favourite house or chair, headland overlooking the sea, a moorland stream etc. It could also be a place entirely of the imagination. Wherever and whatever it is let it be totally for you – your special place that can be private to you whenever you wish. You can become so familiar with it that when you visualise it you not only sense and feel it you can almost touch and smell it.

As you become adept with your relaxation gradually introduce this positive visual image when you are deeply relaxing – and rest in that place which can become a wellspring of nourishment to your inner being. You can also use this very well when you wish to *recall* that state of deep relaxation.

Use your imagination and visualise

Visualisation can be used however you wish. The following are a few suggestions.

- If you are undergoing medical treatment of any kind you can use the power of your imagination to visualise it working in the best possible way for your total wellbeing. Visualise the positive aspects of it rather than dwelling on any negative reaction.

- If you are having difficulty in relating with someone in particular, then visualise yourself and that person communicating freely, openly and honestly. Do this repeatedly until it begins to work and break down previous barriers. Do not be tempted to manipulate a situation just to your own advantage and to someone else's disadvantage as it may well backfire on you. Be positive and well-meaning for both of you so creating a warm relaxed environment for the best possible communication to take place. This is particularly helpful when seeking forgiveness and to forgive.

- If you have a car and wish to park in a crowded area in order to keep an appointment then before you set out to do so visualise a space for you and your car where you can park easily. Visualise parking your car there. Hold that image firmly in your imagination. As you prepare to go to town periodically remind yourself of the image you have created. You may be quite delighted when you get there to find that there *is* a space for you – *especially for you*. Do not be surprised if someone else drives away from a place leaving it clear just as you arrive for you have programmed the situation. Do not be put off if there is no place for you – just accept the situation and continue to practise the visualisation at other times until you begin to strike lucky. Gradually you will begin to create a pattern as you become more and more successful at it.

Several of my students have been doing this for some time with great success – manipulating the traffic is the best possible way to get to classes!

- Visualise yourself:

making decisions easily	forgiving and healing old hurts
making requests	being forgiven for old hurts
refusing requests	in vibrant health with life-force coursing
communicating well	through your veins
freely expressing your emotions	

- Visualise friends and family happy and well.

If there is anyone that you know who is unwell then visualise them in a state of good health. Avoid visualising them unwell. If there is anyone that you know who is near to death visualise them dying peacefully.

Once you start to have success with your visualisation you will have confidence to continue and be delighted with this everyday magic. When your visualisation begins to materialise then fully recognise and acknowledge that it is happening or that it has taken place. This is an important part of its continuation.

Be clear
Be positive
Have good intent
Believe it to be so

When it begins to happen fully acknowledge it. Believe in the power of your imagination to create a better world.

Letting Go

The symptoms of stress are not always apparent at the time of the pressure. In letting go physically and mentally stress often appears and this is why there is so much illness at weekends, on holiday and particularly at Christmas.

One of the best and healthiest things that you can do for yourself is to 'let go' in order to be free and unencumbered by your own limitations. There is a constant pull between 'holding onto' and 'letting go of' that is experienced physically in tight tense muscles, materially with possessions that have served their purpose, mentally with fixed ideas and emotionally with other people who you may want to be free of.

The more you hold onto possessions, people and pleasurable experience the more of a hold they begin to have upon you – they absolutely demand attention. It is very healthy to periodically clear out unwanted possessions that have become an unused hoard, unappreciated and often forgotten. Give them away or sell them if you do not have time to love and cherish them. Feel the releasing effect this can have.

In the practice of relaxation the suggestion is to 'let go' physically and mentally. The effects can be felt immediately as the body and mind begin to feel lighter. Although this appears to be very simple it is also most profound for everything that has ever been experienced is somewhere in the body and mind. Therefore in 'letting go' instead of 'holding on' you may sometimes be overcome with feelings of great joy or sorrow. You may recognise what it is and yet you may not. Whatever it is, you are being offered a golden opportunity to accept what you have been holding onto and to take the opportunity of observing it at a safe distance instead of being caught up in it and then to consider letting it go.

Thoughts and feelings of joy and sorrow may 'well up' and come to the surface. As Kahlil Gibran puts it in *The Prophet*, 'The joy is your sorrow unmasked.'

Aim to accept this in its totality as part of your experience and *feel* it maybe through your laughter and tears. *Of course* it can be painful – that is why it has been pushed away and kept down out of the way so effectively and it has taken such force to do so. The body is effectively dealing with what has been held down by the mind and is now working effectively to keep you healthy.

Forgiveness

In working with relaxation more deeply one of the most predominant features that has come to the fore over and over again has been the theme of forgiveness. Harbouring a grudge can be felt physically, mentally and emotionally and can be the source of a great deal of unhappiness, stress and illness and can prevent you from getting on with your life. *Forgiving is letting go of negative harmful emotions and of punishing yourself and others* with cynicism, doubt, anger, resentment, remorse and condemnation. *Forgiveness is a key factor in the practical everyday principles of health and progress.*

Negative feelings are often masked very effectively with smoke screens of blame, anger, overactivity, 'It's nothing to do with me,' 'see if I care' and as children 'Sticks and stones will break my bones but words will never hurt me' attitude, and so on. 'I can forgive but never forget' is a worn-out phrase that turns on itself for if you truly choose to hold on to the memory *that well* you are partly choosing to hold on to the lack of forgiveness.

In the ancient teachings the suggestion is to prepare for death in the heart of life – to pass on unburdened, uncluttered and with the mind set upon the Divine. To 'tidy up your affairs' usually refers to leaving the practical details in good order for those who are left to deal with them. The same expression can be used for clearing up all that is past and to say 'I am sorry' 'I forgive you' 'I love you' 'Thank you' 'Peace be with you', and all said in love with the tongue residing in the heart.

Even when near to death the fear of dying can be so great that it keeps people alive and holding on for grim death and this is often related to past hurt and a fear of letting go. Therefore seek out opportunities *whenever you can* to clear up your life *now – as you go along*. If it is too difficult to face the situation person to person or if it is too far in the past and you are separated by death or distance then you can constructively use the relaxation, affirmation and visualisation techniques to great benefit.

When deeply relaxed visualise a warm loving environment where you can talk with people from the past and present – do not rush it.

'I let go all past hurt'	*'I let go all that is past'*
'I let go all with love'	*'I forgive you for . . .'*
'I forgive and release myself from . . .'	*'I am free – you are free'.*

If it is too difficult for you to forgive yourself and others for whatever it is then ask God to forgive – give it over to Him and be free. In seeking to release the past hurt you may find that it is just you alone who has been carrying the load all the time and this just highlights the futility of an un*forgiving* nature that is *most* harmful to the person who cannot forgive others and themselves.

In working in this way you may notice that where there has been resentment there is an easiness; where there has been harshness there may be softness – and so on. *Accept that your visualisation and good intent is working well for you.*

It does not matter how physically fit and beautiful you are, how mentally clear and astute you are, if you are not free to let go and love.

What is it all about?

What started out as a straightforward logical approach to stress has developed into a further quest. Physical and mental techniques, eating well, breathing well, moving well and relaxation are nothing if there is no inner stillness. All this activity is an outer attempt to acquire an inner stillness but there will be no stillness and peace if we want to overcome or cope with stress in order to continue in the same frame of reference.

Good health, wealth, love and peace stem from an organic wellspring and love of life – something that stirs deep within – a resonance of vibration with the source of life. In all this activity we can so easily overlook the simplicity of stillness.

In masking the stress we could lose access to our most creative force and spiritual energy. It is the experience of the one that gives access to the other at its height and depth. This is seen as courage in time of difficulty and in the way that great artists, musicians and poets can touch your very soul from their own insight and vast depth of experience.

Create the environment – take time, make time, find time and *just sit and be still*. What could be more simple? When the environment is conducive the stillness 'arrives' unbidden because it wants to be there. After a while you will recognise this to be your lifeblood – the source of your quiet.

> *'Quiet I bear within me.*
> *I bear within myself*
> *Forces to make me strong . . .*
> *. . . And I will feel the quiet*
> *Pouring through all my being . . .*
> *. . . To find within myself*
> *The source of strength,*
> *The strength of inner quiet.'*
> (Rudolf Steiner *Verses and Meditations*)

Ancient philosophy tells us – do not interfere – for if left alone things return to their first principle of natural Divine law and order. We in our sophisticated and civilised world lose touch and forget the simplicity.

Meditation

People who meditate are explorers of their own inner worlds climbing their own Himalayas within and plumbing depths hitherto untapped. Ancient Greek philosophy displays this as an immortal key for above the temple at Delphi are the words 'Man know thyself and thou shalt know God and the universe'.

Stillness is the starting point where we can also reclaim our natural innocence and sense of wonder and experience ourselves and the oneness of things as if for the first time.

> *'We shall not cease from exploration*
> *and the end of all our exploring*
> *will be to arrive back where we started*
> *and know the place for the first time.'*

(T.S. Eliot)

And to conclude, for those who have read to the end, in the classic words of the lovely Buddhist meditation of Loving Kindess:

> 'May you be well
> 'May you be happy
> 'May all things go right for you.'

Physiology of stress

The two main body systems of interest are the nervous system and the endocrine gland system which are very closely interconnected for the control and co-ordination of all activities of the body. The centre of control of the endocrine and autonomic nervous system is the *hypothalamus* which is stimulated by all other parts of the brain. It has nervous connections from all parts of the brain and has specialised groups of neurons which secrete hormones. The hypothalamus is part of the limbic system and as such is also important in directing emotional behaviour. Its role is to interpret perception through experience and send the appropriate messages on through the system.

The nervous system consists of the sense organs, nerves and central nervous system. The sense organs of the eyes, nose, ears, tongue and skin perceive change and send impulses along nerves to the central nervous system. They are like the look-out posts that report any perceived change back to base. The action is then determined and further impulses are sent out along other nerves to organs that will respond appropriately.

The autonomic nervous system is on the course of some of the cranial nerves and is a chain of ganglia interlinked either side of the spinal cord. The activity of the autonomic nervous system is involuntary and below the level of consciousness and its control originates in the hypothalamus. It controls involuntary action of smooth muscles in the body, cardiac muscle and secretions of exocrine glands e.g. digestive and sweat glands. The two parts within the autonomic nervous system are the *sympathetic nervous system* which prepares for action and exerts an active effect and the *parasympathetic nervous system* which exerts a passive effect – both working to achieve balance and harmony through their complementary activities.

The endocrine gland system is a broadcast network of ductless glands that secrete minute amounts of hormones directly into the blood stream: *endo* – within; *crine* – to secrete. The balance of the secretion of hormones is essential for good health, growth and development and a very delicate balance is required between all the various hormones to ensure that all vital processes are carried out harmoniously. Any imbalance can affect intelligence, behaviour and personality. Only a small amount of hormone is released into the blood stream but it can have a most powerful effect. As nerve endings do not extend into cells, chemical regulation within cells is stimulated, controlled and co-ordinated by these *hormones* which are known as chemical messengers. *Hormones* (from the Greek – to excite, to stimulate) are produced in the endocrine glands or groups of cells and are transported in the blood to exert their effects elsewhere in the body.

There are a number of *endocrine glands* in key parts of the body.

Thalamus – considered as a relay centre connecting the hypothalamus with other brain centres.

Hypothalamus – situated immediately above the pituitary and almost at the middle of the brain.

Pineal body – resembles pine cone in shape and projects from the roof and hind part of the brain above the cerebellum.

Pituitary – suspended from hypothalamus by pituitary stalk.

Thyroid – in front of the neck close to the larynx and trachea.

Parathyroid – on the back surfaces behind the thyroid.

Thymus – just behind the breast bone above the heart.

Adrenals – just above and slightly in front of each kidney.

Pancreas – pearshaped affecting stomach and liver.

The *Sex glands* differ in men and women.

Ovaries in women – one on each side of the abdominal cavity, laterally placed. Just beneath the upper rim of the pelvic girdle.

Testes in men – as a foetus, in the abdominal cavity gradually moving down as development takes place until they finally enter a sac (scrotum) just before birth – outside the body.

Whereas the sex glands play an important role in *species* preservation the adrenals are more concerned with the preservation of the *individual*.

The glands of most interest in the study of stress are the **hypothalamus, pituitary** and **adrenal** glands. Some of the nerves in the hypothalamus secrete hormones which feed into the complex circulation system of blood vessels in the *pituitary* gland which itself makes and secretes hormones in response to the releasing factor from the hypothalamus and these are the hormones that move out in the main blood circulation to control other glands like the thyroid, adrenals and ovaries/testes. The *pituitary* gland consists of two separate glands attached to the base of the brain by the same stalk. The two lobes secrete at least six different hormones, one of which is adrenocorticotrophic (ACTH). Increased hormones can be stimulated by external environment e.g. being stuck in a lift, being faced with an angry bull, the sight and smell of food, psychological and emotional stress – and yet there is no direct link between our senses and glands. The messages arrive at the pituitary from the hypothalamus.

The body has a rhythm of deep sleep, waking up, action, intense activity, growth, repair, maturity, decay – all depending for their control on hormones that regulate activities of many different systems in the body.

Like the nervous system, hormones carry signals from one part of the body to another. Whereas nerve signals are electrical and over in a fraction of a second, hormones are chemical messengers in the blood which are active as long as they remain in circulation. The hormones have a deeper, more profound effect upon the body.

Messages carried by the hormones are changing all the time as the needs of the body change – a brilliant supply and demand system e.g. there is a time to eat, sleep, walk, run, work, play etc. Hormones are at work all the time. They help to control many of the body's unconscious activities, particularly those that take place over a long period of time. Each hormone carries a different message for cells somewhere else in the body. A message as specific as 'change pace', 'prepare for action', 'go' and 'stop' – just like traffic lights. Hormones affect a *target cell* – a receptor. Although the hormones travel throughout the bloodstream and all cells are visited by them not all cells pick up the message – only the particular target cells will receive the message which in turn effects a change.

The body is like a finely tuned orchestra and when it plays in harmony it is a source of inspiration to itself, the individual players, the audience and the whole environment. When some of the members of the orchestra are not playing well the whole orchestra suffers – has to adapt – and so it is with the body. The pituitary, known as the master gland, is just like the conductor of an orchestra and organises the complex symphony of the body's daily activities.

The *adrenal* glands are situated on top of the kidneys (hence adrenal). Each gland consists of two completely different glands wrapped around each other and, apart from their close physical proximity, they have very little to do with each other.

The *medulla* (marrow – inner part) produces *adrenalin* which gives the psychological experience associated with fear, and *noradrenalin* associated with anger. The secretion of these two hormones is controlled by the hypothalamus and both hormones produce dramatic changes in the body in response to fear, shock and stress. Adrenalin increases the heart beat and output. Noradrenalin encourages the contraction of small blood vessels in the skin and abdominal viscera so that more blood is circulated to the voluntary muscles. The hormones are secreted after the gland is stimulated through the nerve fibre of the sympathetic nervous system and this causes rapid preparation of the body for swift action. These two hormones are associated with the fright, fight or flight syndrome.

The *cortex* (rind – outer part) releases glucocorticoids and mineralocorticoids for tissue repair, androgens and oestrogens which are concerned with masculine and feminine qualities. Sections of the cortex are controlled by ACTH which is secreted by the front section of the pituitary gland. The amount of ACTH is determined by the amount of cortex secretion in the blood. Corticoids regulate a large number of important bodily functions including regulation of the metabolism of carbohydrates and proteins, regulation of the amount of mineral salts and water, reduction of inflammation, determination of female sex characteristics. *Target cells* for adrenalin are all over the body e.g. heart muscle which is affected by contracting with more force and at a higher rate.

Relax without tranquillisers

Chemical insulation is no substitute for life even though drugs are often used in an attempt to solve a wide range of problems. Tranquillisers may well have a place in medicine as they can alleviate a great deal of pain and suffering but control and guidance is essential. Tranquillisers dull the perception, slow down reaction and can leave you feeling dull, heavy, apathetic, irritable, aggressive and depressed. They can produce a separation between you and the source of your anxiety – it does not go away – it is only masked. Often the tranquillisers themselves lead to bigger problems.

Minor tranquillisers

In the 1960s the minor tranquillisers were introduced to replace the barbiturates as an apparently 'safe' sedative with fewer side effects and said to be non-addictive and not dangerous in overdose. Previously, in reducing these tranquillisers it was thought that the original anxiety still existed and so the drug was continued. However, in time and with further study it became apparent that these were side effects. The drugs were producing the effect.

The minor tranquillisers of the benzodiazepine family include valium, ativan, librium, mogadon, dalmaine, serenid D, serenid forte. Their specific names include diazepam, lorazepam, chlordiazepoxide, nitrazepam and oxazepam. This information refers to minor tranquillisers of the benzodiazepine family and not major tranquillisers or anti-depressants.

Research now shows that these drugs are only effective as tranquillisers for up to four months maximum and as sleeping pills from between three to twelve days. The side effects include drowsiness, stuttering, dry mouth, unsteadiness, clumsiness, weight loss and gain, loss of muscle co-ordination, giddiness and blurred vision.

STOP BEFORE YOU 'POP'

If you are considering tranquillisers please stop to ask yourself the questions:

What is the real problem here?

Is there another way of coping with it?

Maybe you have identified the source of one or several problems that require attention, if so –

Is it something that can be changed?

Can you seek out an impartial friend who is prepared to truly listen?

Listening is one of the best therapies. Is there a trained counsellor or support group in your area? The library, citizens advice bureau, doctor and health centres may be able to put you in touch with someone.

Ten pointers

1 Do not take tranquillisers unless you really need them.

2 If you do decide to start take as small a dose as possible.

3 Take them for as short a time as possible.

4 Never increase the dose beyond your prescription.

5 If you already take tranquillisers report to your doctor at regular intervals. Do not rely upon repeat prescriptions. This is your responsibility. Ask to be monitored and remind yourself and your doctor of the original reason for wanting the drug in the first place. Circumstances may have changed. Be honest with yourself and your doctor. How is he going to know these things unless you tell him? When he is writing out a prescription tell him about any other drugs that you are taking.

6 *Always check your prescription.* There may be an increase or decrease – if so, ask why? – *This is your responsibility.*

7 *Never lend or give pills* to other people and *never borrow* or *take pills* from other people.

8 Do not take minor tranquillisers *if you are pregnant,* a *nursing mother, very elderly* or a *heavy drinker.* Alcohol should not be taken when using tranquillisers or anti-histamine or travel pills. Due to their drowsy effect it is inadvisable to drive or operate heavy machinery whilst under the influence of these drugs.

9 *Make a list of all the things that you enjoy* and make you feel life is worth living and then make a list of all the things that are undesirable to you. *How can you expose yourself to more of the first list* and less of the second? Can you *change your attitude* to any on the second list?

10 *Make a list of your problems.* If reducing tranquillisers is one of them put it near the top. Once you have dealt with the reduction of pills you could be much stronger and more able to cope with the other set of problems.

Preparation for reduction

Stage I

Imagine yourself coping without tranquillisers and have a clear visual image of yourself with improved memory, coordination, clear thinking, feeling love and happiness. Have this vision of yourself within the not-too-distant future. Expect to succeed. Promise yourself a brighter future. Take the chapter *Help Yourself to Health* very seriously. Become familiar with relaxation techniques in the *Relax and Unwind* chapter.

This will increase your confidence to carry on. Have the relaxation techniques well established before you start to reduce your tablets.

Plan of action

You will need a notepad.

1 In the beginning write down why you want to cut down your tranquillisers and recall the original reason for starting them. Keep writing and writing and periodically stop to ask yourself the question 'Why is that?' . . . 'Why is that?' . . . This simple but powerful technique may unleash root causes of your distress. You could also draw or paint your anxiety, problem or tranquillisers – this could be very revealing to you. Keep all these things as a record to look back on.

2 Talk to your friends and family and explain what you are planning to do.

3 See you doctor and tell him what you would like to do and ask for his co-operation and support. Aim to establish a good working relationship with your doctor and tell him that you need time. Many doctors are very sympathetic to this difficulty and will give you the support for which you are asking. If you think it appropriate then take this book along so that the doctor knows what your intentions are. Refer to the cassette tape *Relax without Tranquillisers.*

Ascertain the following information:

- the size of the dose and the strength of the tablet in milligrams
- how long you have been taking them
- whether you are taking other drugs
- the kind of support available to you.

Refer to the illustration as an example and set out a similar table across a double page of your notepad using the same headings. Start a fresh page every time you make the slightest reduction.

Stage II – Cutting down and putting the plan into action

Reduction of the dose must be gradual as there can be severe reactions. A rough guide is to allow one month for every year that you have taken tranquillisers. The higher the dose the longer you may need to come off. Targets are helpful guidelines but can produce their own stress so have a plan and be prepared to adapt and change it depending on how you are dealing with the situation at the time.

Do not be hasty – take time.

Do not stop your tranquillisers suddenly – phase them out.

Do not stop every other day or even one day a week – gradual, even reduction is essential.

Do not keep lowering and raising the dose – establish your plan and stick to it.

Ask your doctor to prescribe the same amount but in smaller doses.

For example 30 × 2 milligram tablets can be prescribed instead of 12 × 5 milligrams. This allows you more scope with cutting down gradually. Here is an example – valium is made in 2, 5 and 10 milligram tablets. If you are taking 3 × 5 milligrams (15 mg total) you could possibly have the prescription changed to 7 × 2 milligrams (14 mg total). You will have already reduced the dose by 1 mg. Stay with this until you feel confident to make further reductions however small.

You could still take them three times daily e.g. 2 × 2 mg. In the morning, 2 × 2 mg. in the afternoon and 3 × 2 mg. in the evening. According to which time of day suits you cut out just a part of the tablets at that time until you feel confident to take the next step – and so on.

You may wish to keep the status quo for a while. However you may reach the stage where you become impatient – then hold on. *Remember what is at stake.* Whatever you decide to do please take each step carefully and with confidence – keep referring to your original aim.

Watch the need when there is extra stress. If you choose to temporarily increase the lowered dose make decisions about how long you anticipate this before returning to the lowered dose. Make no hard and fast rules here as these can prevent your progress.

PLAN OF ACTION (THIS IS ONLY AN EXAMPLE)				
PRESENT DOSE OF TRANQUILLISERS	REACTION	HOW I FEEL	ACTION TO TAKE	PROPOSED NEXT STEP
Step One				
15 mg valium (3x5 mg)	Dizzy, not really here – as though I am somewhere else.	Numb	1. Start to take charge somehow. Ask for help. 2. Go out into the fresh air more. 3. Talk to someone about how awful I feel. 4. Try the relaxation.	1. Have a really good walk for 15 minutes every day. 2. Find a good friend or counsellor who will help on a regular basis. 3. Listen to the tape on relaxation and see if it helps – give it time. 4. Make an appointment to see doctor to ask for his/her help.
Step Two				
14 mg valium (7x2 mg)	Quite pleased with myself. Had a really good cry and felt better. Still feel hazy but feel more as though I am taking over rather than being taken over.	Scared, nervous and angry but have to continue.	1. Continue with fresh air, relaxing and talking with a friend. 2. See doctor again to see how things are going, not necessarily to decrease any further yet. 3. Dare I think about sorting out things at work? Shall I tell my partner why I am so upset?	1. Walk and Treat* for at least $\frac{1}{2}$ hour every day. 2. Talk with colleagues at work. 3. Talk with partner. I really need to talk.

*See passage entitled TREAT in 'Help Yourself to Health', chapter 5.

LIVERPOOL
JOHN MOORES UNIVERSITY
AVRIL ROBARTS LRC
TEL. 0151 231 4022

Stage III – Withdrawal

As you reduce the dose sounds may appear louder, sight clearer and brighter, taste buds sharper, touch more acute and smell stronger. This can be quite alarming to begin with but it will subside.

Emotions come to the surface and you may become restless, want to cry, shake, be angry or talk incessantly. These are natural reactions to the suppression. Dreams could become more vivid. If you suffer from insomnia please refer to the cassette tape *Relax and Sleep Well.*

You may also experience signs of flu – aches, pains, sweat, sneeze, cramp, hallucinations, fatigue, sleepiness, irritability, headaches, forgetfulness and a desire for the drugs. Crying can be a healthy part of the healing process.

Keep on keeping on and expect the best not the worst. Not everyone experiences withdrawal symptoms.

Know that you are not alone – thousands of other people are fighting back against drug dependence. Do not blame yourself or anyone else. This is a waste of your valuable vitality and you need all the positive energy you can muster to deal with this situation. Accept the situation as it is and make decisions as you adjust carefully and start to achieve. You may feel a lot worse because the body is sending messages that you need the drugs and you may find all sorts of excuses for going back to the old dose. You may temporarily feel a little better if you go back but you will have reverted and have to start again. If you are fortunate enough to have found a self-help or support group tell them how horrid you feel. Feeling ill can be a sign of recovery. Please do not revert back – keep on keeping on. Continue to write in your book – particularly your reactions, how you feel and actions to take. Continue the daily practise of relaxation exercises. Regularly refer to suggestions in the chapters *Help yourself to health* and *Creative living*. Keep a visual image of yourself free from pills. Postpone new responsibilities and major decisions at this time. Recognise that some days are easier than others and live one day at a time reviewing each day as you go. Really look around you instead of trying to get through the day as quickly as possible. Train yourself to think how much good it is doing you. If you are preparing a meal – prepare it totally. If you are driving – drive. If you are reading a book – read it – and so on. Whatever you are doing do it totally – just for five minutes, just for ten minutes, just for one hour. This is a mental trick that has helped thousands of people to break a habit.

You may find that thoughts and emotions return from the past and you may be able to deal with them now with a different attitude. The original reason for taking tranquillisers may well re-appear. Do not start to panic but treat this as an opportunity to deal with it in a different way.

Stage IV – Relief without drugs

Take one day at a time. Let the past go, let the future take care of itself. Just take one day at a time rather than a lifetime. Refer to the passage entitled *Choices* in chapter four. Look at your lifestyle – are there changes you wish to make? Put your needs first. This may appear foreign to you but it is important to treat yourself as a most valuable person. Learn to live with anxiety. Beware of external pressure from other people who may prefer you to be quieter and less reactive. They may wish to encourage you to go back on tranquillisers – anything to keep the peace. It can be hard for the people around you too – after all the change can be very threatening.

Affirmations

I choose to live and experience life
I am in charge of my life
I love myself unconditionally.

Relax and sleep well

Lack of sleep is not always harmful and not sleeping does not always mean that there is a sleep problem. However, the anxiety that accompanies the lack of sleep can produce a problem. Physical discomfort, illness, worry, fear, depression, boredom can be the cause of insomnia *and* of sleeping too much. Chronic insomnia is usually a symptom of an underlying cause.

Sleeping pills

The first stages of sleep are a non-dreaming state and the brain waves become slower. During this time the body engages in repair, growth and replenishing and there are powerful forces that work toward the healing process. The dream state then follows when rapid eye movement occurs known as the REM phase. This ideally takes about 25% of the total sleep time and is concerned with maintenance of the mind. Sleep then lightens before deepening again.

Even though sleeping pills can be necessary in extreme conditions they usually have their side effects of disrupting the natural rhythm and reducing the REM phase of dreaming. This in itself can become a problem. If you take sleeping pills already and wish to reduce them or do without them altogether then please do this very gradually and carefully seeking advice and support. Also refer to the section entitled *Relax without Tranquillisers* for reduction of medication.

Accept, adjust and achieve

If the cause of your sleeplessness is known then you could ask yourself if it is something that can be dealt with. Can anything about it be changed? If it is impossible to change the situation then aim to accept it. Your attitude to the situation is the key.

How much sleep

Quality of sleep rather than quantity is the aim. Requirement of sleep varies and the average is between six and eight hours. Trying to sleep beyond your need can be fruitless and negative. Tossing and turning in bed in order to get the last out of the time spent there can produce an irritable 'getting out on the wrong side' syndrome. Why not just simply get up and use the time well?

Being awake during the night can be beneficial. Make a warm drink, read a good book, write letters, enjoy a creative activity like drawing, painting or relaxation exercises and meditation – and enjoy it all rather than thinking that you should be asleep. *Trying* to keep your eyes open can, in fact, lead to closing them.

Bedtime

Honey is well known for its soothing healing effect. Try a teaspoon or more in either warm water, warm milk, diluted pure grape juice or camomile tea. Tea, coffee and cocoa contain caffeine and act as a stimulant. These drinks also work as a diuretic which may lead to waking to go to the toilet.

Water has a very therapeutic effect. Cold water over the back of the neck can help to take the heat out of the day. A warm bath can be a comfort and conducive to 'washing away the day' and resting.

Relaxation and exercise

Sleep and relaxation are both required although there are physiological differences. Many people who regularly practise deep relaxation and meditation require less sleep due to the deeper levels of rest achieved during the day. Learn the trio of neuro-muscular relaxation, complete deep relaxation and solar breathing in the chapter *Relax and Unwind*.

Develop and dissolve

Develop positive attitudes of sleep and let the negative attitudes of 'not enough sleep' dissolve. Develop the attitude of 'If I fall asleep that is wonderful' and 'If I do not fall asleep that is wonderful'. *If at first you do not succeed* then *give up trying* for it could be the trying that keeps you from sleep. Let it come, let it go, just drift in and out of sleep in your time and rhythm.

'Instead of counting sheep talk to The Shepherd'.

Affirmation

All the sleep that I really need is coming to me now to refresh and revitalize.

Anxiety attack, panic and hyperventilation

What is it?

'Help, I want to get out' 'Help, I can't get out'. Head swims, heart races; sweat profusely; choking; having a heart attack? Having a stroke? Going to die? Losing consciousness?

But NO – the body is behaving as though it is facing real danger for no apparent reason. Please know that this is not unusual – you are not alone. Many many people have these horrible attacks.

Hyperventilation is when you breathe too shallow and too quick. This pattern is linked to the 'fight or flight' response which prepares the body for high activity in the face of danger.

Why does it happen?

Sometimes this happens for no apparent reason but it could be triggered by many different things including a deep recognition of a fearful situation and not succeeding.

When does it happen?

It can occur anywhere, whether in a crowded place or alone or even first thing in the morning upon waking. It can produce a vicious circle as the fear of an attack may well bring one on.

What to do?

Look after yourself, eat well, breathe well, exercise well and learn to relax.

Use the relaxation and breathing exercises as groundwork. Avoid drugs as they only bring temporary relief and mask the problem which may well return when off the drugs. It is you who needs to be in control of yourself and not the drugs. Ask other people for help and confront your fear. If you know that crowded places bring on an attack ask a friend to be your 'minder'.

When you are feeling in control you could rehearse and deliberately seek out a situation that causes the panic or just breathe fast and shallow. If this produces an attack then practise the first aid treatment set out below and remain in charge.

First aid treatment

1 First remind yourself of the 'recall' in the chapter *Relax and Unwind*. Take up the stance as suggested – upright spine and open chest whether you are standing or sitting. Remember the position with the thumbs and forefingers to remind you of the state of relaxation.

2 Say simply to yourself – *Stop!*

3 Take a slow deep breath into the base of your lungs, hold onto that breath for a moment and thoroughly exhale as you say to yourself – *let go*.

4 Wait a moment before you breathe in deeply again slowly and evenly. Hold onto the breath for a moment and then exhale slowly as you repeat once more to yourself – *let go*. Repeat the breathing pattern until you begin to feel more in control of the situation.

5 Fix your gaze on something you can become familiar with, for example a tree, plant or flower out of the window, or a pleasant picture or even a tiny crack in the wall – anything on which you can truly concentrate whilst you breathe deeply. Remind yourself who you are, where you live and where you are at the time.

6 Begin to experience the panic as a wave that washes over you and that *when you decide* it will leave you.

Extra tips

1 If you have access to a toilet then go and sit there and practise your deep breathing and, as you exhale bear down, and really let go.

2 Splash your face with cold water.

3 Place a cold, wet flannel over the bridge of your nose and cheekbones.

4 Breathe into a *paper* bag (not plastic or polythene). Practise this beforehand.

Know that the stage will pass – learn to live with it and it will eventually leave you, particularly when your attitude towards it has shifted. Stay put, let it flow through and over you. Running away or out of the room does not get rid of it as you take it with you. Be brave and ride it out.

Basic sitting position

Sit either on a chair or the floor. In choosing a chair aim for upright support. In choosing the floor try different positions with the legs – kneeling, legs crossed or straight and outstretched. The main aim is an upright and comfortable spine whereby the chest can be open and the breathing uninhibited by a sunken chest. It is good to experiment and find the position that really suits you – maybe two or three different positions.

Sit tall with the head well balanced on top of the spine and the chin very slightly tucked in in order to ease the back of the neck. Avoid jutting the chin forward and compressing the back of the neck.

If sitting on a chair have your feet flat on the floor.

Rest the hands – *either* in the lap cupping the back of the left hand in the palm of the right *or* palms of the hands flat on the thighs *or* resting on the knees, whichever is appropriate for the position that you have chosen.

Close your eyes and prepare to relax.

Sit tall and feel the uprightness from the base of the spine up through the back of the waist, in between the shoulder blades and the back of the neck.

Breathe in and feel as though you are being drawn up like a puppet with a string attached to the very top of your head. As you breathe out just run the attention down over the body relaxing but without slumping.

Do this several times in preparation for the exercises.

Basic lying down position

Lie flat on the floor on a rug or mat.

Look down the length of your body and have your legs about twelve to eighteen inches apart so that when the toes turn in towards each other they do not quite touch.

If the lower back is uncomfortable in this position then *either* bend your knees having feet flat on the floor resting the knees against each other; *or* place a cushion under your knees; *or* rest your legs and feet on a few cushions, the side of a low sofa or chair.

Have your arms about ten inches away from the trunk with the palms of the hands turned uppermost.

If for any reason it is inappropriate to have your head flat on the floor then use cushions to support the head and neck.

Roll your head from side to side and then let it rest centrally as you tuck the chin in slightly in order to lengthen the back of the neck.

Close your eyes and prepare to relax.

Getting up from the floor

It is very important to take care when getting up from the floor particularly if you have been lying there for a while. Doing so without care and in a rush can undo all the good work of back stretching and relaxation.

1 Push your heels away and rotate your ankles and feet, stretch your arms up and behind and have a really good s-t-r-e-t-c-h.

2 Rub the palms of the hands together and place them over your closed eyes. Open your eyes behind your palms, then close them again. Release the hands and open your eyes wide, look around and prepare to sit up.

3 Place the palms of the hands flat on the floor underneath the back of the waist and feel the contact of the floor with your elbows.

4 Raise the head, take a deep breath in, push down on your hands and elbows and carefully sit up.

Benson MD, Herbert, *Beyond the Relaxation Response* (Collins)

Bhagavad-gita, (Penguin Classic, translated by Juan Mascaro)

Birkinshaw, Elsye, *Think Slim – Be Slim* (Thorsons)

Caddy, Eileen, *Opening Doors Within* (Findhorn Press)

Coleman, Dr Vernon, *Women and Tranquillisers* (Corgi)

Cott, Allan, *Fasting: The Ultimate Diet* (Bantam Books)

Cousins, Norman, *Anatomy of an Illness* (Bantam Books)

Diamond, Harvey and Marilyn, *Fit for Life* (Bantam Books)

Dominian, Jack, *Depression* (Fontana)

Ferucci, Piero, *What We May Be: Visions and Techniques of Psychosynthesis* (Turnstone Press)

Gawain, Shakti, *Creative Visualisation* (New World Library)

– – *Living in the Light* (Eden Grove Editions)

Gibran, Khalil, *The Prophet* (Heinemann)

Grant, Doris and Jean Joice, *Food Combining for Health: New Look at the Hay System* (Thorsons)

Hambly, Dr Kenneth, *Overcoming Tension* (Sheldon Press)

Hanson, Dr Peter, *The Joy of Stress* (Pan)

Hanssen, Maurice, *E for Additives* (Thorsons)

Harrison, John, *Love Your Disease it's keeping you healthy* (Angus & Robertson)

Hay, Louise, *You Can Heal Your Life* (Eden Grove Editions)

Hewitt, James, *Meditation* (Hodder & Stoughton)

– – *Relaxation* (Hodder & Stoughton)

Jampolsky MD, Gerald, *Love is Letting Go of Fear* (Bantam Books)

Kenton, Leslie, *The Biogenic Diet* (Arrow)

Kenton, Leslie and Susannah, *Raw Energy* (Arrow)

Kirsta, Alix, *The Book of Stress Survival* (Unwin)

Krishnamurti, Jiddu, *Meditations* (Victor Gollancz)

Mulford, Prentice *Thought Forces* (G. Bell & Son)

Orbach, Susie, *Fat is a Feminine Issue* (Hamlyn)

Patanjali, *How to Know God: Yoga Sutras of Patanjali* Translated from Sanskrit by S. Prabhavananda & C. Isherwood (Vedanta Press)

Pietroni, Dr Patrick, *Holistic Living* (Dent)

LIVERPOOL
JOHN MOORES UNIVERSITY
AVRIL ROBARTS LRC
TEL. 0151 231 4022

Plato, *Republic* (Penguin Classic) Translated by Desmond Lee

The Quiet Mind (White Eagle Publishing)

Riley, Vera, *Positive Living* (R. S. Trade Press)

Selye, Hans, *Stress and Distress* (Corgi)

Silva, José and Philip Miele, *The Silva Mind Control Method* (Granada)

Still Voice: Book of Meditation (White Eagle Publishing)

Treasury of Devotion Ed. Arthur Russell (Arthur James Ltd)

Trine, Ralph Waldo, *In Tune with the Infinite* (Bell & Hyman)

Tyrer, Dr P., *How to Cope with Stress* (Sheldon Press)

van Lysebeth, Andre, *Pranayama – the Yoga of Breathing* (Unwin)

Further Listening

Mind Your Body Cassettes

A series of cassette tapes prepared to complement the content of the book. This is a way of sharing to encourage a sensitive communication between mind, body and spirit leading to improved health and sense of wellbeing. Each manuscript is written and professionally recorded by Jenni Adams and her soothing voice carefully guides the listener through each tape.

Relaxation

'If you let go a little you will have a little peace
'If you let go a lot you will have a lot of peace
'If you let go completely you will know complete peace and freedom
'Your struggles with the world will have come to an end'

(Achaan Chah)

RELAX AND UNWIND   R1
Relax, Let go, Be Still . . .
Simple and brief – once learned never forgotten!
Straightforward and to the point – ideal for busy people.
Used extensively in business, clinics and hospitals.
Fifteen minute sitting relaxation

JUST RELAX   R2
That's all – heed the soothing suggestion and guidance to rest deeply for twenty minutes with tranquil music accompaniment. A gentle, easy tape.

CREATIVE RELAXATION   R3
Let go and release unnecessary tensions to encourage a sense of stillness. Two relaxations –
Awareness of the breath (sitting); Creative visualisation (lying down)
Used by many on a regular basis to help relieve stressful conditions.

Self-help guides

'The same mind that drags you down can also pull you up'

(Ernest Wood)

POSITIVE LIVING
G1

Themes and affirmations to dwell upon and gradually build an accumulative effect to gain confidence, strength and inner peace.

Based on the old adage –

'That which is nourished grows

'That which is not nourished fades and dies'

THE BREATH AS A KEY
G2

Stress, anxiety and chest complaints can all be helped by the restoration of 'right breathing'. The breath is a key to physical vitality, mental clarity, emotional stability and spiritual awareness. Here is a detailed, balanced programme of breathing and relaxation exercises based on Yoga instruction and simplified for safe application.

RELAX AND SLEEP WELL
G3

The root of sleeplessness is often to be found during the day although it manifests in the quiet of the night.

Light exercise for the body and deep relaxation for the mind gently lead the listener to enjoy natural rhythmic sleep with soothing music accompaniment.

RELAX WITHOUT TRANQUILLISERS
G4

Natural tranquillity and equilibrium can often be found in the recesses of a relaxed mind.

This is an informative tape with deep relaxation and gently guides the individual with great care and encouragement to cope without tranquillisers wherever possible. Used extensively and in clinics.

Exercise

'Are you as young as your spine?'

Practical, informative, balanced programmes with clear commentary to encourage suppleness, strength and stamina.

Set out in order of progression. Illustrations on inset covers.

RISE AND SHINE   E1

Wake up and ease your way into the day with gentle music and exercise. A good introduction and 'warm up' to be used at any time to thoroughly stretch the body – lying on bed or floor.

Carpé Diem – Grasp the Day!

RELAX AND MOVE GENTLY   E2

It's never too late to bend! This is particularly designed for people with restricted or limited movement whether of a temporary or more permanent nature as the programme is chosen to maintain and improve suppleness and breathing capacity. Sitting on a chair for exercise and relaxation.

STRETCH, BREATHE AND RELAX   E3

A lovely routine to complement the next two titles – standing, kneeling and lying flat. Includes Egyptian *Salutation to the Sun* and closes with deep breathing and relaxation.

RELAX YOUR MIND AND BODY   E4

Good all-round exercise sitting, standing, kneeling and lying flat. The second side provides four different relaxation exercises. Each side can be used independently.

The very first tape and still one of the most popular!

S-T-R-E-T-C-H FOR LIFE   E5

A more challenging s-t-r-e-t-c-h programme – lying, kneeling, standing. Includes Link Movements of Chest-Expansion and The Bridge – closing with deep relaxation.

Yoga

'Yoga is the control of thought-waves in the mind'

(The Sutras of Patanjali I)

Yoga practice is a harmonious set of exercises essentially working with the body and mind. Five programmes set out in order of progression and to complement each other. Clear instructions with benefits and effects given throughout. Encouragement is given to develop at your own pace. Illustrations on inset covers.

YOGA FOR FITNESS   YI

Ideal as an introduction. The whole of the first side is devoted to clear explanation of the celebrated *Salutation to the Sun.*
Side Two includes seven particular postures to complement and finishes with relaxation.
Each side can be used independently.

BEFRIEND YOUR ARTHRITIS   Y2

This is a good all-round programme for anyone wishing to keep supple. It is specifically for people with arthritis and aims to restore harmony and ease away stiffness and pain. Focus on legs, hips, neck, wrists, shoulders and balance. Includes fourteen postures, two link-movements, Pranayama (expansion and awareness of breath), Deep Relaxation and Visualisation.

HATHA YOGA PRACTICE   Y3

Complete classic programme known as the Rishikesh sequence. Includes Surya Namaskar (Salutation to the Sun); fifteen asanas (postures), Relaxation, Pranayama and Meditation.

OPEN UP TO YOGA   Y4

Reference is made to the Eight Limbs of Yoga and the Chakras (wheels of energy). The programme of postures is based on the seven nodal points of the body – opening and closing – and ends with Deep Relaxation and Pranayama.
Used as a teaching module by some Yoga establishments.

YOGA NIDRA   Y5

Nidra means 'sleep'. This is a deep relaxation – a classic practice where physical sensation is reduced, circulation increases and the mind expands in order to experience the 'oneness' of things. This is a very expansive and uplifting experience – to be used at any time and especially to aid the healing process.

Meditation

'Meditation does not create perfection; it allows perfection to disclose itself by removing the obstacles to its realization'

(Hari Prasad Shastri)

The first side of each tape in this series is a clear narrative. The second side gives guidance into the meditation. Suitable for individual and group use.

MEDITATION MADE EASY   MI

Ideal introduction that aims to remove the shroud of mystery that often masks the simplicity of meditation. The focus of this quiet meditation is the awareness of breath – chosen for its subtlety and ease.

MEDITATION FOR PEACE   M2

An inner journey of discovery through a talk on peace as a state of mind rather than something that exists outside ourselves. The meditation begins with the focus of peace within – then expands the awareness to outer things – and returns to a deep inner peace.

'Better than a thousand useless words is one single word that gives peace'

(Dhammapada 8)

INNER SILENCE   M3

A particular and definite process to slow down thought and quieten the mind – ideal for the busy intellect. Five stages carefully lead the listener to inner silence. Based on the age old classic Yoga practice Antar Mouna (inner silence)

CONTEMPLATIVE MEDITATION   M4

To contemplate is to enter into your own inner room – the secret chamber of your heart. In order to do this various mantras are mentioned but this particular meditation is based on the gift from the Psalmist *'Be Still and Know That I Am God'*

A TIME TO FORGIVE   M5

Harbouring a grudge or a feeling of guilt can be at the core of a great deal of unhappiness, stress and illness and can prevent us from getting on with our lives. Forgiveness is therefore a practical everyday principle of health, harmony and progress.

The guided meditation includes using the imagination to visualise – asking for grace and strength to forgive others and ourselves. A visit to Taizé Community in France – a place of love and reconciliation – gave birth to this tape.

Just imagine

The imagination is immensely powerful and mainly responsible for how we live our lives. This series will help to harness that power and use it positively for happiness, healing and joy.

SECRET GARDEN   J1

Here is an opportunity to put things into perspective, to see patterns emerging in life and to live in the present moment – to release the past with its regrets, longing and clinging and release the future with its worries and excitement – and to truly live in the moment – HERE AND NOW – unadorned and without attachment.

So take a journey into your own secret garden – a place to rest and re-charge

LAKE OF TRANQUILLITY   J2

Water has long been known as an ancient symbol of the soul. Let it be a source of nourishment on every level – body, mind and spirit. Two guided journeys – the lake at sunrise and at sunset – a lovely way to start and end the day. Deeply restful.

Music accompaniment – 'Watercolours' by Anthea Gomez

CITY OF LIGHT   J3

Here we are drawn to the Light.

Side One – a candle meditation to focus the outer gaze, aid concentration and induce a deep calm.

Side Two – carefully leads the listener to a place of light within themselves – returning feeling lighter and uplifted. (Music accompaniment – *'Sounds Relaxing'*)

> *'There is a Light that shines beyond all things on earth, beyond us all, beyond the heavens, beyond the highest, the very highest heavens. This is the Light that shines in our heart'*

(Chandogya Upanishad)

Music

SOUNDS RELAXING S1

Soothing music to create a relaxed atmosphere – a gentle ebb and flow. Ideal for a restful background whether at work, rest or play.

Total playing time 80 minutes.

Created 'with a little help from my friends'

(Roger Fordham and Roger Messer)

Index

acceptance: *vs* change 23
adaptation: and stress 9–11, 19
additives, food 79–80
adrenal glands 5, 132, 133
affirmations 39–41
   for breathing 70
alcohol, use of 48
allergies, food 80
animals: and relaxation 48, 108
anxiety attacks 140–2
attitudes: to problems 22, 23, 50–1

balance: in life 8, 9
Bhagavad-gita 20, 74, 75
Blake, William 73
body awareness: in relaxation
   115–18
body language 85
brain/brain waves 106–7
breathing 57, 59–61, 70
   in exercise routines 89
   exercises 61–70
   in relaxation 112–13
   solar 123–4
bulls, angry 3, 4, 8

change: in life 18–19, 22
   vs acceptance 23
   see also life-changes
Charles, Prince 15
chewing 82–3
choices, making 41–4, 75
Christoph, Friedrich 23
communication, importance of
   35–6
companions, choosing 49
coping 20–1, 25
cost: of stress 1
Coué, Emile 39
Cousins, Norman 49–50
creativity: and emotions 53–6
cycles, individual 31–2

decision-making 29, 38
diaphragm: in breathing 60
   exercises 62–4

diet(s): and nutrition 76, 77
disassociation, conscious 115–18

eating habits, improving 78–9,
   81–3
Ecclesiastes 31
effects: of stress 5–8, 11
Eliot, T.S. 130
emotions, expressing 51–6
endocrine gland system 131–3
environment
   internal/external 9, 82
   and life-force 58–9
   and stress 18–19, 20
exercise(s)
   breathing 61–70
   on conscious choice 42–4
   on current situation 12–13,
      32–3
   on life-changes/future 28, 33
   physical 87–103
   for posture 86
   relaxation 109–26
expectations: of life 39
eyes, exercises for 99–101

fasting 80–1
fat, meaning of 72–3
Faulkner, Kim 55
feelings, expressing 51–6
feet/legs: exercise 97
'fight or flight' 2–5
   and hyperventilation 61, 140
   vs relaxation response 105, 106
food 71–83
forgiveness 127–8
'fourfold remedy' (Patanjali) 44–5
Fuller, Buckminster 48

Gibran, Kahlil 36, 127
gratitude 50–1
grief 52
Grossinger, Richard 21

hands, exercises for 101–3
Haynes, Jim 48

helping others 53
Holmes, Thomas 25–6
hormones 5, 131, 132–3
humour, sense of 49–50
'hurry sickness' 9, 61
hyperventilation 61, 140
hypothalamus (gland) 131, 132

illness: as coping 13–14, 21
imagination: in visualisation 124–6
   via solar breathing 123–4
immune system 25
indecision 29, 38
information: overload 28–9
ions: in atmosphere 57–8

James, William 20, 29
jaw, exercises for 101

koshas (bodies) 14

laughter 49–50
learning: in life 18, 21
letting go 53, 126–7
life-changes 4, 8, 25–6
   anticipating 26–7, 28
life-force 57, 58–9, 76
   recharging: exercise 69–70
lifestyle: under stress 7–8, 18
loneliness 50
losing: *vs* letting go 53
lungs: and life-force 58, 59
lying down: basic position 142–3

Mark: Gospel 20
Masefield, John 30
massage 49, 102–3
meditation 130

neck, exercises for 98
nervous system 5, 32, 131
neuro-muscular relaxation 119–21
ninety minutes: cycles 32
nose/nostrils 32, 59, 62
   breathing exercise 68–9
nourishment (food) 71–83

office routine: exercises 89, 93–7
overeating 74, 78, 79
overstimulation 2, 26

panic attacks 140–2
Patanjali 14, 45, 60
'people poisoning' 30
physiology: of stress 3–4, 131–3
pituitary gland 132
Plato 14, 25
posture 85–6
prana *see* life-force
problems, attitudes to 22, 23,
    50–1
proxemics 29–30

Rahe, Richard 25–6
reactions: to stress 2, 5–8
    see also 'fight or flight'
recall: of relaxed state 114
relaxation 17, 105–6, 107, 108
    effects 109, 110
    techniques 109–26
requests, making/refusing 36–8
respiration *see* breathing

rhythms, natural 30–1
rituals, value of 27–8

Salutation to the Sun 88, 89–93
Schweitzer, Albert 49
Selye, Hans 1
shoulders, exercises for 98–9
sitting: basic position 142
skin: and life-force 58, 59
sleep problems 11, 139–40
smiling 49
smoking 48
solar breathing 123–4
solar plexus: in exercises 69–70,
    124
space, personal 29–30
'special needs' exercises 89, 98–103
Steiner, Rudolf 129
stillness 31, 129, 130
    in breathing 60–1, 113
    in relaxation 108, 113
stressors 1–2
    life-changes as 4, 8, 25–6
structure: in life 29
substance, quality of 9, 10

success: and failure 20
sunshine, value of 48, 100
symptoms: *vs* cause 13–15

Thoreau, Henry 32
time management 30–3
tolerance levels 9–13
Tonegawa, Susuma 25
tongue: and life-force 59, 82
touch, importance of 48–9
tranquillisers 48, 133–5
    programme to reduce 135–9
treats 50
'trio': of relaxation exercises
    118–24

under-stimulation 12
Upanishads 22

visualisation 124–6
    in solar breathing 123–4

waiting: and stillness 31
'wake up' exercises 88, 89–93
work: and leisure 32–3, 47–8

If so wished the following can be photocopied and used as an order form

Cassettes £7.95 each – Any 2 or more £7.50 each

RELAXATION		Quantity	Amount
Relax and Unwind	R1		
Just Relax	R2		
Creative Relaxation	R3		
SELF-HELP GUIDES			
Positive Living	G1		
The Breath as a Key	G2		
Relax and Sleep Well	G3		
Relax without Tranquillisers	G4		
EXERCISES			
Rise and Shine	E1		
Relax and Move Gently	E2		
Stretch, Breathe and Relax	E3		
Relax Your Mind and Body	E4		
S-T-R-E-T-C-H for Life	E5		
YOGA			
Yoga for Fitness	Y1		
Befriend your Arthritis	Y2		
Hatha Yoga Practice	Y3		
Open up to Yoga	Y4		
Yoga Nidra	Y5		
MEDITATION			
Meditation Made Easy	M1		
Meditation for Peace	M2		
Inner Silence	M3		
Contemplative Meditation	M4		
A Time to Forgive	M5		
JUST IMAGINE			
Secret Garden	J1		
Lake of Tranquillity	J2		
City of Light	J3		
MUSIC			
Sounds Relaxing	S1		
	Total required		
UK Postage, packing, handling			£1.50
EUROPE AND OVERSEAS POSTAGE – *STERLING ONLY PLEASE*			
EUROPE Postage, packing, handling			£2.25
OVERSEAS Postage, packing, handling			£3.00
	TOTAL		£

Orders despatched promptly but allow up to 21 days delivery. If dissatsified return within 21 days of receipt, giving reasons for replacement or refund. Please complete BOTH SECTIONS IN BLOCK LETTERS as one will be used for posting your order to you.

Cheques payable to JENNI ADAMS

    MIND YOUR BODY CASSETTES

    5 THURLOW ROAD

    TORQUAY, DEVON TQ1 3DZ

Name.. Name ....

Address .... Address ....

....

...............................Post Code ....Post Code ....

LIVERPOOL
JOHN MOORES UNIVERSITY
AVRIL ROBARTS LRC
TEL. 0151 231 4022